TRUCKERS GUIDE TO HEALTH AND LONGEVITY

TRUCKERS GUIDE TO HEALTH AND LONGEVITY

SUSAN ASHLEY, MD

To order additional copies of this book, contact:
Xlibris
1-888-795-4274
www.Xlibris.com
Orders@Xlibris.com
762054

CONTENTS

SECTION THREE

NUTRITION

SECTION FOUR

ALTERNATIVE MEDICINE

SECTION FIVE

SUPPLEMENTS AND EXERCISE

SECTION SIX

SUCCESS

Introduction

Imagine that you are a truck driver. You get up at 4:00 AM to be on the road by 4:30. You slept in the cab of your truck, which is your home for three weeks of the month. Breakfast is a fast-food egg sandwich or burrito washed down with coffee. You use the public toilets at the truck stop, wash up quickly, and hit the road by 4:30. It's still dark out, but the highways are already busy with other drivers just like yourself. Now it's time to drive for the next ten to twelve hours on the road.

Your food is fast-food, and over the years, your belly has gotten bigger. You find yourself winded more easily than you used to with loading and unloading. With the last DOT exam, the doctor only passed you for one year because of the high blood pressure that has developed over the years. The large varicose veins have become more painful, and you find yourself tired all the time. Frequent heartburn is a common problem, and you have to take pills for that every day. You've been offered nothing that could help from the medical world. Nothing, that is, until now. Now things are about to change—changes that will allow you to get your life back.

This book is written for a forgotten population that our society depends on and for an industry that employs over twelve million people in every city and town in the US. Truck driving is one of the deadliest occupations in the country, with 745 drivers killed in 2016.

But even more importantly, truckers face a much higher risk of chronic illness, including obesity, high blood pressure, sleep apnea, diabetes, and physical inactivity. Truck drivers are absolutely essential for our nation's economy, yet their health issues have been largely ignored. And now a recent study is out, showing that commercial truck drivers with three or more medical conditions *double to quadruple* their chance for being involved in a crash compared to their heathier counterparts.

If you're reading this book thinking that you're going to get typical medical advice, like eat low fat, use margarine instead of butter, and take your statin drugs for cholesterol, you'll be either happily surprised or sadly disappointed. The health of our society, and especially among our truck drivers, is progressively worsening, and for the first time in human history, our children may not live longer than their parents. In this book, you will learn what you can do to take control of your health and add years to your life, giving you back the energy and vitality you had when younger.

The advice of the traditional medical establishment is slanted toward using pharmaceutical drugs for every condition and symptom instead of getting to the root cause of the problem. While I am a medical doctor, traditionally trained with a board certification in family medicine, after twenty years of practice, I went back to school and obtained a second board certification in antiaging and regenerative medicine. This is where I learned to look at things completely differently and learned how to use supplements and nutrients to reverse disease and many other modalities that are considered alternative medicine.

For example, you will learn

- the true cause of heart disease, which is *not* cholesterol, and how to slash your risks;
- why statin drugs for cholesterol should rarely be prescribed and why they may be harmful for you;

- butter, whole milk, eggs, and nuts are not only *good for you* but encouraged;
- how to *reverse* diabetes, sleep apnea, and high blood pressure so your DOT can be extended back to two years instead of one;
- why drugs for heartburn, taken chronically, will dramatically increase your risk of dementia, osteoporosis, and heart disease and how to get off these drugs and heal the stomach;
- how you can effectively lose weight once and for all with a diet that doesn't leave you hungry and is best for lowering cholesterol, blood sugar, and insulin and is *not* low-fat;
- how bioidentical hormones—testosterone for men and estrogen for women—can help you regain motivation, vitality, muscle mass, and libido while slowing the aging process;
- why testosterone not only does *not* cause prostate cancer but also actually reduces the risk of prostate cancer;
- the best exercise program for truckers to reduce fat, gain muscle, and lose weight and can be done in the least amount of time; and
- how antiaging therapies can be incorporated into your routine to turn back the hands of time, including the newest research on stem cell therapy.

If you are a truck driver who is interested in learning how to prevent and/or treat the many maladies that plague this occupation and how to pass your DOT every time, you've come to the right place. This book is for you, and I hold nothing back.

Section One

COMMON HEALTH PROBLEMS

Chapter 1

THE TRUCKING INDUSTRY

Watch, listen, and learn. You can't know it all yourself. Anyone who thinks they do is destined for mediocrity.

—Donald J. Trump

At any given time, there are 2.5 million long-haul trucks on the road. The trucking industry employs five million truckers, with another twelve million people employed in supporting the trucking business. Our national economy depends heavily on truckers delivering their hauls throughout the US, Canada, and even Mexico. I can't think of a single industry that doesn't depend on truckers, and the adage "If you bought it, a truck driver brought it" is never so true. Whether it's retail, construction, hospitals, gas stations, groceries, raw goods, or oil, all depend on trucks to distribute cargo necessary for their industry. Your job is an honorable one, one on which our society is completely dependent, and can provide a good living for your family.

However, the health of our truck drivers is deteriorating, and they face many health risks because of their occupation.

As a physician, I see truck drivers from all over the country—some drive locally and many are over-the-road (OTR). Certified to perform

Department of Transportation (DOT) physicals, I've noted over the years that my trucker patients have greater health problems than the general public. This not only affects their livelihood but also reduces their longevity and quality of life.

The following are some examples of actual patients, with names changed of course.

Tim is forty-six and has been driving for twenty-two years. He's gone for three weeks, home for four days, then off again. Over the years, his weight has gone from 180 to 268 pounds, and he now has type 2 diabetes that's controlled on oral meds, with high blood pressure. These limit his DOT exam to once a year rather than two years. Because of the stricter federal guidelines by the Federal Motor Carrier Safety Administration, we've had to screen him for sleep apnea, which he has; and he requires treatment. He's developed chronic swelling of his legs and numbness and tingling of his feet, which often impair his sleep. His energy and motivation are much lower than it used to be, and he finds that he gets short of breath easily with even light exertion.

Jack is fifty-five and has been driving since his twenties. His weight has increased nearly a hundred pounds to 290 pounds, and he also has developed the triad—diabetes, high blood pressure, and high cholesterol. Sleep apnea is thrown in the mix, and thankfully, he does tolerate a CPAP. But he despises it, wondering if there are any alternatives that would still allow him to treat this condition. His family is completely dependent on his ability to be on the road to make a living, and he's worried that his health will cut his career short. He's also developed COPD, or emphysema from smoking, and is trying to cut back. His doctor says he's a walking heart attack waiting to happen, but he feels powerless to change.

Sarah is forty-nine and has driven for fifteen years. She is a local driver, so she can be home at night with the kids. Her weight has increased forty pounds over the years, and she's developed chronic low-back pain and joint stiffness. Having gone through menopause last year, she is having constant hot flashes and night sweats and does not sleep well, never feeling rested. She is always fatigued, can't get rid of the belly fat, and has lost the enthusiasm and spark of life she used to have. Last year, she developed a DVT or deep venous thrombosis of the leg, a blood clot on her leg, and had to be on blood thinners for six months. This has left her with chronic swelling in the leg, and she's worried that she'll develop another one that could not only end her career but also be life-threatening.

I have many other patients just like these, and I've been frustrated with how to help, other than to say the usual "Exercise, lose weight, and quit smoking." This advice has not worked for my patients, and I had to come up with a different strategy—a comprehensive plan on what could be done to change their lives, optimize their health, and regain vitality.

This book is written from an antiaging medicine perspective, with advice not found in the traditional Western medicine world. Antiaging medicine is the newest and most exciting field of medicine! I am geared to find the root cause of disease to reverse the condition, instead of writing a prescription for every symptom, and improve the quality of life and extend the lifespan. Practicing antiaging medicine has given my patients the best chance at success in optimizing their health and the best chance at completely reversing all the conditions mentioned above.

Did it work for these patients? Tim has lost sixty pounds and is no longer diabetic. His blood pressure is normal, and he's put the CPAP on the shelf. He exercises regularly, even when driving eleven hours a day, and has energy and enthusiasm again.

Jack has quit smoking and has started to reverse the damage done to his lungs from the thirty-year habit. He's lost fifty-five pounds and is continuing to lose more. Sleep apnea and diabetes are things of the past, and he was given a clean bill of health on his most recent physical.

Sarah has learned what dietary changes are needed to completely resolve the joint pain and is off the daily ibuprofen. She's lost thirty pounds and has joined a regular exercise class. Bioidentical hormones have completely stopped the hot flashes, and she feels like she has been given her life back.

It can be done, and it starts with you!

Chapter 2

HEALTH PROBLEMS OF TRUCKERS

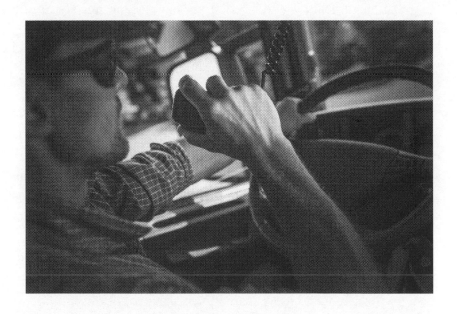

The greatest danger for most of us is not that our aim is too high and we miss it, but that it is too low and we reach it.

—Michelangelo

The "National Survey of US Long-Haul Truck Driver Health and Injury" study done in 2014 showed a common set of problems associated with the trucking industry. The study intended to focus on long-haul truck drivers, who seem to have the most problems. The most common health issues for truckers are the following:

- *Obesity.* Truck drivers are twice as likely to be obese as the rest of the US population, with 69% of truckers being obese and 17% of them being morbidly obese. In comparison, one-third of the US adult working population are obese—7% morbidly. Transportation workers are the fattest and have the highest risk for chronic health problems of any occupational group. Obesity is defined as a BMI of 30 to 39; morbidly obese is a BMI of more than 40. The obvious reason? Sitting for long stretches at a time and eating food at truck stops, often unhealthy and fried. Excessive snacking, stemming from boredom on the road, contributes.

- *Hypertension or high blood pressure.* This is usually related to excessive weight, aging, and genetics.

- *Diabetes, type 2.* There's an epidemic of diabetes in the US because of the obesity epidemic. Drivers can now continue driving as long as their diabetes is controlled; a waiver is needed if you're on insulin.

- *Smoking.* The prevalence of smoking in truckers is more than double the US population—51% versus 17%. This contributes to a number of diseases, such as chronic cough, COPD (emphysema), asthma, earlier heart disease, and lung cancer.

- *Sleep apnea.* A third of truckers are now diagnosed with obstructive sleep apnea, and it is projected that this number will increase to more than 50% because of obesity.

- *Heart disease.* This is one of the most devastating diseases to affect the drivers. Truck drivers are especially at risk for heart attacks. The long hours of sitting, lack of exercise, obesity, poor diet, diabetes, and high blood pressure all contribute to the increased heart disease risk.

- *Blood clots.* A clot can occur in the legs, where a piece can then break off and travel to the lungs, causing a blood clot to the lungs or a pulmonary embolism. This can be life-threatening and needs immediate treatment. Drivers are more susceptible to clots because of the long periods of immobility.

- *GERD.* This means gastroesophageal reflux disease or, in other words, heartburn. Why is heartburn such a big deal? Because the meds used to treat reflux, known as PPIs. It should not be taken for longer than two weeks at a time. If taken long-term, they are associated with many devastating side effects, such as dementia, stroke, heart disease, increased risk of infection, protein deficiency, and osteoporosis. These drugs include Prilosec, Nexium, Protonix, and Prevacid (the purple pill).

- *Joint and back pain.* This plagues many drivers, especially after prolonged sitting for hours on end and lifting heavy loads.

In addition, truckers, like any other population of aging adults, suffer problems such as menopause, declining testosterone, loss of muscle mass, flabbiness, brain fog, depression, insomnia, and lack of energy.

Reading this, it could be easy to become depressed, but don't be! If you're new to truck driving and don't have any health problems yet, I will show you how to prevent them from occurring in the first place. And if you've been driving for many years and have one or more of the conditions above, I'll show you how to potentially reverse each of these and get your life back. Don't listen to doctors or friends that say your diabetes can't be reversed or that you'll never get off your blood pressure medication. I've been in practice for twenty-five years, and I see it done every day.

Chapter 3

DIABETES

Every day is a second chance.

We'll address diabetes first because it has reached epidemic proportions in our society and in the trucking community. There is a 50% higher occurrence of diabetes in truckers than the national average. It has become so prevalent that some trucking companies have hired diabetes coaches to help manage their disease, and it has become one of the largest challenges to health-care systems.

The cost of diabetes annually is more than $100 billion in the US, and the average health-care costs for a diabetic are $12,000. Diabetes causes leg amputation, kidney failure, blindness, ulcer, heart disease, and stroke; and it significantly increases the risk of developing cancer. And it can shorten your life by ten to fifteen years.

What is diabetes?

There are two types. Type 1 DM occurs mostly in childhood where the immune system destroys the pancreas. The pancreas is an organ that lies behind the stomach and makes digestive enzymes and insulin. Type 1 DM must be treated with insulin; there is no other option at this time. In the future, type 1 DM will be cured with stem cell transplants, but that is down the road. Those with type 1 DM cannot obtain a DOT.

Type 2 DM is the type of DM we're talking about, and for our purposes, this is what we will focus on. Type 2 DM is the type associated with weight gain around the abdomen. The belly fat, otherwise known as the middle-aged spread or beer belly, is extremely hazardous for our health, and the fat surrounds our organs in the abdomen. Think of gel-like globs of fat wrapped around our liver, kidneys, and pancreas. This type of fat is called *visceral* fat, and it is *vicious*! It is biologically active, making its own hormones to ensure the cell's survival while creating inflammation throughout our body. This visceral fat is so inflammatory that it can stress all our organs, increasing inflammation within our arteries, which increases risk of heart disease.

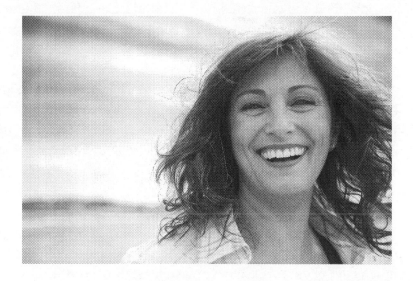

The abdominal fat causes insulin resistance, which means the pancreas is making insulin, but the body's liver and muscle cells aren't responding to it as they should. Insulin is the hormone that manages blood sugar and brings sugar levels down after you eat. Foods that are higher in sugar (desserts, carbs, pasta, and potatoes) cause more insulin to be secreted than foods higher in protein and/or fat.

When we eat, our food is absorbed and broken down into simple sugar called glucose or fructose. This enters our bloodstream and sounds an alarm, causing insulin to be secreted in response. The insulin allows the sugar to enter our cells to be utilized as energy, such as in muscle cells, brain cells, etc.

But when there's too much glucose in our blood and our cells don't need any more, then it gets stored as fat. The process is extremely efficient since in caveman times, we never knew when our next meal would come, and we needed to store the fuel to call upon later. Now, of course, this is rarely needed, and we just keep on storing it. That's why insulin is known as the fat-storing hormone.

The process occurs more quickly with refined carbs, such as white bread, rice, junk food, alcohol, and sugary foods. These foods are rapidly absorbed and converted into sugar, releasing large amounts of insulin, needing to put the sugar somewhere, having nowhere to go but storage as fat.

The average American eats over ten pounds of sugar each month or 4½ cups per week! Refined sugar is 99.7% pure calories—no vitamins, minerals, or proteins, just carbohydrates. Therefore, 20% of the daily caloric intake of every American is spent on a refined food that has no nutritional value and that plays havoc on the body's chemistries.

And with type 2 DM, the insulin is not used properly. This is called insulin resistance. To make up for it, the pancreas makes more insulin. Eventually, it can't keep up, and blood sugar starts to rise. That's why people with T2DM have high blood sugar and high insulin.

Symptoms of DM include the following:

- *Fatigu*e. This is very common, but of course, there are about one hundred different causes of fatigue. However, high blood sugar in the bloodstream means the cells are being starved of sugar, which makes you more tired and irritable.

- *Excessive thirst and urination.* The excess sugar can pull fluid from your tissues. This makes you thirsty. You drink more, then you urinate more. This is not good when you're driving for a living.
- *Constant hunger.* When there isn't enough insulin, your cells aren't getting enough sugar inside the cell, which triggers intense hunger.
- *Blurred vision.* High blood sugar levels can change the shape of the lens in your eyes, causing blurring of vision.
- *Numbness of feet.* The high blood sugar can affect the nerves in your feet, causing tingling, numbness or pain.
- *Poor wound healing.* DM decreases healing rates and can increase risk of infections.
- *Darkened skin.* There's a condition some people get with DM—patches of dark velvety skin in the folds and creases of the body, like the armpits and neck. This is called acanthosis nigrans, and it signals insulin resistance.

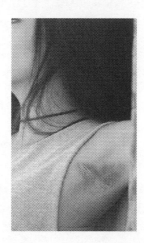

- *Gestational diabetes or DM in pregnancy.* This occurs in 4% of all pregnancies. A third to a half of women with gestational DM will develop type 2 DM within five to ten years after childbirth.

The most important thing to know about T2DM is that it can be reversed—completely reversed! And by reversing DM, you will dramatically lower your risk of heart disease, kidney failure, stroke, and cancer!

Why are truck drivers at such risk of DM? Because of the hours of inactivity sitting behind the wheel and the tendency to eat too many carbs, junk food, and fast food. We're going to change all that and turn your life around!

How do doctors diagnose diabetes?

There are two ways: one with blood sugar levels and another with something called an A1C or glycated hemoglobin.

Normal fasting blood sugar should be less than 100. So if your fasting blood sugar or glucose is 101, it's abnormal. But what we really should know is that fasting blood glucose should not be over 85. Anything more than 85 indicates that insulin resistance is already occurring. The ADA says a fasting sugar of 99 is normal, but in reality, this can actually double your risk of heart disease. A fasting sugar of 85 or higher will increase risk of heart disease and stroke; in reality, the cutoff should be 83.

Fasting means twelve hours without food and nothing to drink but water.

What we've confused is *normal* with *common*. Just because something is common does not mean it's normal or, certainly, optimal for our health. I teach my patients to not only pay attention to the *abnormal* values on labs but also the *optimal* values. An optimal fasting blood sugar is *83 or less*.

Another way to diagnose DM is a glucose tolerance test. It is a perfectly horrible test, whereby a person who is fasting then has to drink seventy-five grams of glucose dissolved in water. It's sickeningly sweet and makes you gag as you choke it down. Then you measure your blood sugar one hour and two hours after finishing the drink. A blood sugar of 140–198 is defined as prediabetes, and one of 199 or greater is diabetes. But this is quite ridiculous, as that means a sugar of 139 is normal but one point later is pre-DM? What about 135? Or how about 198? And no one wants to choke the drink down. If I'm considering doing this test, I'll tell a patient to fast. We'll draw the blood sugar, then go out and eat a high sugar/carb meal—such as pancakes with syrup, orange juice, and fruit—then come back one hour and two hours later for repeat blood sugar. It's a much more enjoyable way of testing!

The next way to diagnose DM is through a blood test called an A1C or glycated hemoglobin. It's actually measuring how much glucose is bound to hemoglobin in red blood cells. Red blood cells are constantly living and dying and then live, on average, for three months. Thus, the A1C gives an indication of your level of blood sugar over the last three months. And it explains why the higher the A1C, the more short of breath you are. If more of your hemoglobin is bound by glucose, there's less to carry oxygen to your tissues.

An A1C level of 6.5 or higher is DM; 5.7–6.4 is defined as pre-DM.

Here's a chart showing the average blood sugar corresponding to A1C:

5—100
6—130
7—160
8—190
9—220

Are A1C levels accurate? For the most part, yes. However, there are conditions that can skew the results. Anemia, where there is less hemoglobin to start with and less, therefore, to bind to glucose, can cause A1C readings to be artificially low. And people with certain conditions such as thalassemia or sickle cell anemia can have inconsistent results. Other causes of a false A1C is either liver or kidney disease. But for most of us, the A1C is an accurate measurement of disease.

Optimal A1C levels are between 4.4 and 5.3. Many studies have shown a direct correlation between high A1C and heart disease. Patients with A1C levels less than 5% had the lowest rates of CVD, and there is a linear increase in CVD as A1C levels increase above 4.6%—a level that corresponds to a fasting blood sugar of 86. Another way of stating this is that the risk of heart disease in people without DM *doubles* for every percentage point increase greater than 4.6%.

The point is, do not wait for your levels to go from normal to pre-DM to early DM and upward to be treated. Start right away. If the A1C is 5.4, treat now and prevent DM from occurring in the first place. And if your doctor has given you the diagnosis of DM, remember, it *can* be reversed, and we will do everything we can to help you!

Treatment of diabetes involves diet, supplements, and/or medications. In the ongoing chapter, we'll discuss in detail the dietary approaches to reverse diabetes. For now, this is just a brief overview.

Cut out the carbs in your diet. What are carbs? Basically, these are foods that are readily converted to sugar by your body. This includes bread, cereal, rice, pasta, potatoes, sugar, pastries, alcohol, and fruits.

The top twenty sources of carbs in the US diet are the following:

- Potatoes
- White bread
- Cold breakfast cereal
- Dark bread
- Orange juice
- Bananas

- White rice
- Pizza
- Pasta
- Muffins
- Fruit punch
- Coca-Cola
- Apples
- Milk
- Pancakes
- Table sugar
- Jam
- Cranberry juice
- French fries
- Candy

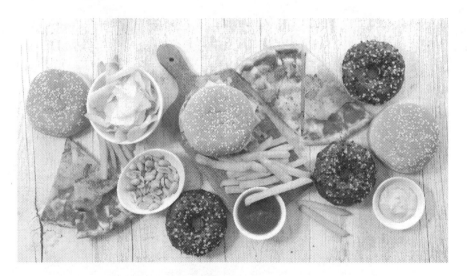

A breakfast of oatmeal, toast, and juice is simply horrible for a diabetic or for anyone over age forty for that matter. It causes so much insulin to be secreted to handle the sugar load that it takes hours for the insulin to come down, all the while trying to store the sugar as fat. Try a breakfast of two eggs, bacon, and coffee with some cream and sweetened with stevia. Or try my favorite, a chocolate peanut butter protein shake with vegetables and berries thrown in.

It's twenty grams of carbs, full of protein and nutrients, easy to make, and delicious!

But like I said, we'll talk about this in a lot more detail. That's coming up in section 3.

Treatment of type 2 DM usually involves medications. The most commonly used drug is called metformin, and it is the best oral drug for DM. It doesn't cause low blood sugar; it helps you lose weight, and it even has antiaging properties to it. There are studies done on patients who smoke, showing it may reduce the risk of lung cancer. However, metformin does cause B12 deficiency, and this must be taken with it. Use sublingual or under-the-tongue drops, as taking B12 in a capsule is not absorbed well.

But the most effective, absolutely best medication for *men only* that you never hear about is . . . testosterone! Any man with type 2 DM is testosterone deficient, and replacing bioidentical testosterone can often provide a complete cure for their DM. This is not discussed in mainstream medicine, but it is widely used in practitioners who practice antiaging medicine. I'll discuss this in much more detail in chapter.

Supplements are very important to our health. I use supplements, vitamins, and nutrients for many conditions; but the most important thing to realize is, they must be high quality and medical or pharmaceutical grade! Most vitamins sold are food-grade vitamins and have very poor absorption and little, if any, of the nutrients on the label.

Supplements for diabetes can be very useful, and I have seen many patients decrease their A1Cs from DM range to pre-DM or from pre-DM to normal. The most common supplement I use is berberine. Berberine has potent anti-inflammatory effects and works like the drug metformin in reducing glucose production by the liver. It also decreases cholesterol and triglycerides and inflammation, particularly something called hs-CRP, a blood marker of inflammation. This level should ideally be less than 1.0. The more abdominal fat you have, typically, the higher the hs-CRP.

Chromium is also important. The more sugar you eat, the more the body increases the excretion of chromium in the urine. Chromium is needed to increase insulin sensitivity, and most diabetics are deficient in chromium. The average dose of chromium picolinate is 400–600 micrograms.

Sugar also increases the elimination of calcium and magnesium and decreases the rate of their absorption. Magnesium deficiency increases insulin resistance. I typically recommend magnesium glycinate, citrate, and/or maleate. The more absorbable forms between 200 and 600 mg per day.

CLA, or conjugate linoleic acid, has been shown to normalize blood sugar and help with insulin resistance. Take 1,000–3,000 mg.

An herb called fenugreek lowers blood sugar due to its high content of soluble fiber, which acts to decrease the rate of stomach emptying, therefore delaying the absorption of glucose from the small intestine. It also helps to lower cholesterol and triglycerides. Because fenugreek is high in fiber, calcium and medications should be taken separately

Gymnema is an herb that lowers blood sugar in both T2DM and T1DM at a dose of 400 mg/day. It can lower blood sugar, A1C, cholesterol, and inflammation.

Fish oil, or the omega-3s, are very important to reduce the risk of heart disease, stroke, dementia, and arthritis. Take between 3,000 and 4,000milligrams per day, and make sure it's been purified. All the mercury and toxins should be removed. Take it with food. You shouldn't burp up fish oil after you take it. If you do, change brands.

Cinnamon, cloves, and bay leaves have the insulin-like activity of lowering blood sugar. Use them in your cooking as much as possible.

In the next chapter, we'll talk about a disease that often occurs with diabetes: high blood pressure or hypertension. They go hand in hand, and where there's one, there's often the other.

Chapter 4

HYPERTENSION

Your future is not set until you invent it.

Julie has driven a truck for fifteen years and is an owner-operator, enjoying the freedom and responsibility that comes with being an owner. However, over the last several years, she's noted that her blood pressure seems to be creeping up, from 110/70 to 132/88 then 144/94 and higher. Her doctor said it was time to be treated, and she knew her DOT exam was coming up, leaving her no choice. But she felt great. Why treat something that wasn't even bothering her and take a drug that might cause side effects?

Blood pressure is something familiar to most of us. We get this checked every time we go to the doctor's office or the dentist, and we can even get it checked at our pharmacy or grocery stores. Many of us have a blood pressure cuff at home, but we don't know what the numbers actually mean.

Blood pressure is the force or pressure of blood as it flows inside our arteries. Systolic BP is the top number and refers to the amount of pressure in your arteries during contraction of the heart. Diastolic BP is the bottom number, referring to your blood pressure when the heart muscle is between beats.

High blood pressure, or hypertension, is known as the silent killer, as it rarely causes any symptoms until a stroke or a heart attack occurs. Headaches associated with blood pressure are relatively rare. Hypertension is the number 1 cause of heart disease in the US, and if you have it in your family, you may have a higher risk genetically.

Can a driver with hypertension keep their CDL? Absolutely, but the blood pressure must be controlled, and they will have to recertify every year rather than every two years.

A driver with a systolic BP of 140–159 and/or a diastolic BP of 90–99 has stage 1 hypertension and may be medically certified to drive for a one-year period. Certification examinations should be done yearly thereafter, and BP should be less than 140/90.

A driver with a BP of 160–179 over 100–109 has stage 2 hypertension and usually requires treatment with antihypertensive medication. The driver is given a one-time certification of three months to reduce the BP to less than 140/90. He or she may then be recertified for one year from the date of the initial exam. The driver is certified annually thereafter.

A driver with a BP of 180/110 or greater has stage 3 hypertension and is disqualified. The driver may not be qualified, even temporarily, until the BP is reduced to 140/90 or less. The driver may then be certified for six months and every six months thereafter, as long as BP remains 140/90 or less.

There are a number of medications used to treat hypertension, and these include the following:

Diuretics. Lower BP by eliminating excessive fluids through urination. These are among the oldest drugs used for BP and are more effective for those that are sensitive to salt intake and for blacks. However, diuretics alone are a poor choice of a medication, as they have not been shown to reduce mortality (risk of death), and they cause insulin resistance, increasing the risk of diabetes. Examples include furosemide (Lasix), hydrochlorothiazide, triamterene, and indapamide (Lozol).

These drugs can be hard for a trucker to take, as they will cause you to stop more often to use the restroom! Common side effects include dehydration and low potassium. Sometimes taking extra potassium is needed. Your doctor will monitor your electrolyte levels.

Beta blockers. These drugs reduce epinephrine or adrenaline, relaxing the heart and, thereby, reducing the amount of blood pumped by the heart. They're often used after a heart attack (myocardial infarction or MI) since studies have shown that taking these drugs for at least one year after an MI can help to prevent a second event.

Side effects with beta blockers are common and include fatigue, the number 1 side effect; reduced exercise capacity; and erectile dysfunction.

Common beta blockers are atenolol, bisoprolol, metoprolol, propranolol, and nadolol.

ACE (angiotensin-converting enzyme) inhibitors. These are drugs that block an enzyme that activates angiotensin, which controls BP within the walls of blood vessels. They help relax blood vessels and help to reduce the amount of water absorbed by the kidneys. They are the most common drugs used for BP control, as they are generally well tolerated, cheap, actually decrease mortality, and preserve kidney function.

Side effects include a dry cough that can develop. I see it in about 5% of my patients. If you get the cough, it usually will not resolve until you discontinue the medication. Other side effects may be a rash and kidney damage. After I start an ACE inhibitor, I'll always check kidney function three weeks later to ensure that the creatinine has not increased. If it has, this could be a sign of the narrowing of the arteries to the kidneys and needs to be evaluated further.

Common ACE inhibitors include lisinopril, enalapril, quinapril, and benazepril. It's anything that ends in a *pril*.

ARB (angiotensin II receptor blockers). These block the hormone called angiotensin II that's responsible for constricting arteries, allowing the blood vessels to relax and widen. They also reduce the amount of water your body retains, which also lowers BP. These drugs are frequently prescribed when an ACE inhibitor has caused a cough.

Side effects are the same as an ACE, except for the cough. Dizziness and headache can occur but infrequently.

Common ARBs include losartan (Cozaar), valsartan (Diovan), and irbesartan (Avapro).

CCB (calcium channel blockers). They prevent the passage of calcium from entering the cells of the heart and blood vessel walls, allowing for greater ease of blood flow and reduction of BP. They're also used to treat heartbeat irregularities such as atrial fibrillation.

Side effects include edema or swollen ankles (common), palpitations, constipation, and dizziness. Actually, every BP med can cause dizziness simply by reducing your BP!

Common CCB meds include amlodipine (Norvasc), diltiazem (Cardizem), felodipine (Plendil), nifedipine (Adalat, Procardia), and verapamil (Calan).

Of these meds, the most commonly used one is amlodipine. I rarely use more than 5 mg because if you increase the dose to 10 mg, the ankle edema is much more likely to occur.

Alpha blockers. These drugs selectively block particular chemicals called alpha-adrenergic receptors that cause arteries to constrict.

Side effects are fairly common and include dizziness but are more pronounced than the other meds, drowsiness, and increased heart rate.

Medications in this class include prazosin (Minipress), terazosin (Hytrin), and doxazosin (Cardura).

I often get asked if there are any supplements or foods that can lower BP so that a medication might not even be needed. There's a great advantage to this for truckers, in that if they can get the BP down naturally, then they can remain on a two-year recertification rather than one year.

There are a number of things you can do to lower BP. First and foremost is weight loss. If you have the spare tire around the abdomen, chances are, losing some of that weight will lower your BP. Even just a ten-pound weight loss can drop the BP enough so that meds are not needed.

Regular aerobic exercise can lower BP significantly, as much as ten to fifteen points on systolic and five to ten points on diastolic. A combination of aerobic and resistance training is best. In upcoming chapters, we'll talk about how to get this accomplished while on the road, even when driving for ten hours a day.

A number of supplements have been shown to lower BP, and I recommend all my patients with hypertension to take at least two of these:

Magnesium. This mineral is responsible for over four hundred enzyme processes throughout the body, and most Americans are deficient in it. Low magnesium can cause muscle cramps, especially the charley horses you get at night. Nocturnal leg cramps are almost always a deficiency of magnesium, then calcium, and thirdly, potassium. Magnesium deficiency can also cause heart palpitations, fatigue, anxiety, and insomnia. The most commonly sold magnesium is magnesium oxide, which is poorly absorbed and frequently causes diarrhea. The best absorbed forms are magnesium glycinate and chelate, and most of us need between 200 and 1,000 mg a day. Milk can decrease BP by providing magnesium, calcium, and potassium.

L-arginine. This has blood pressure–lowering benefits and promotes the health of the lining of our blood vessels. It is the building block of NO, or nitrogen oxide, production. It will make your arteries more flexible and improve blood flow to the heart, improving congestive heart failure.

In men, L-arginine will increase not only the blood flow to the heart but also the blood flow to the arteries that supply blood into the penis, helping to achieve an erection. Viagra works similarly by increasing the production of NO to improve arterial blood flow. Viagra, interestingly, was first made as a drug for patients with heart disease; erectile dysfunction improvement was found as a much-desired side effect.

What is the typical dose? Most supplements provide 500 mg per capsule. Taken orally, arginine is absorbed rapidly and broken down even more so, with most of it gone in less than one hour. What is needed is a sustained release formula, which is available but is quite expensive. We've been able to contract with a company to make it much more affordable. It's taken as three tablets twice a day. I've been using this product for some time now with hypertensive patients and have seen it lower the BP from 156/100 to 124/72; 142/98 to 126/70; 158/98 to 136/86. These are just some examples, and as you can see, this is as much as any drug.

Vitamin D. If there is only one vitamin that you take that can have the most profound impact on your health, it's vitamin D. You'll see me talk about this vitamin frequently as it is so important. Not only does it enhance your immune system to make you more resistant to disease but it also lowers risk of cancer, heart disease, osteoporosis, and lowers blood pressure.

No matter where you live, you're likely low in D, and your levels need to be between 70 and 90. Do *not* accept a normal of 30. A minimum of 40 is needed just to protect the bones from osteoporosis. We need to focus on what is optimal, not what is normal. Normal levels, as cited by labs, is comparing yourself to sick people, which we don't want to do. We want to strive for optimal levels, and for most of us, that means we'll need to take between 2,500 IU and 10,000 IU per day. Take more in the winter since we do get some D from sunshine. Where we live, in the northwest, we rarely see sun in the winter, and I take 10,000 a day until June, when I back off to 10,000 every other day until October. D is best absorbed with oil or fat, so take it with your meal. Make sure your D is D3, not D2, which is not as well absorbed.

Potassium. If you have normal kidney function, you likely won't need to take potassium or K. However, the average American diet is low in K, and this can contribute to a higher BP. You can get a five-point reduction in eating K-rich foods, such as, in order of highest to lowest, avocadoes, acorn squash, spinach, sweet potatoes, salmons, dried apricots, pomegranates, coconut water, white beans, and bananas. An optimal K level in the blood is at least 4; if your level is less than 4, it may be *normal* but not optimal. It will increase your risk of heart failure and heart arrhythmia.

Protein. Numerous studies have shown that high protein intake reduces BP. This does not, however, include cured meat like, sadly, bacon. Daily intake recommended is 1.0–1.5 g/kg/day. This formula is used to convert pounds to kilograms: 1 lb. × 0.453 = kg. So for a two hundred-pound man, it would be $200 \times 0.453 = 90$ kg. Or for a simpler way to figure it out in your head, just divide your weight by two and subtract a little.

It's not only meat. Whey protein at 20 g a day has been shown to significantly reduce BP by 8/5 mm Hg in four weeks. The whey must be hydrolyzed to be effective. This is rich in bioactive peptides.

Vitamin C. Doses of 500 to 1,000 mg twice a day are needed to drop systolic BP by 3.6–17 mm Hg. It also has the effect of making certain BP meds more effective, such as calcium channel blockers.

Flavonoids. There are over four thousand flavonoids, which are biologically active, colorful plant compounds that occur in fruits, vegetables, and certain herbs and are powerful antioxidants. Not only do they help prevent cancer, but they also cause dilation of arteries and prevent atherosclerosis or the buildup of plaque.

Different flavonoids include fruits; green, red, purple, and yellow vegetables; green tea; and dark chocolate and cocoa. Dark chocolate is *not* a milky way. This is sugar-laden milk chocolate with none of the health benefits. Eat a diet that is full of the colorful vegetables and fruits, especially dark berries, pomegranates, and green leafy salads.

CoQ10. This a nutrient found in every muscle cell in the body, and it is especially critical in the heart and brain. As we age, we make less CoQ10, and our levels go down, contributing to fatigue, muscle wasting, and brain fog. If you take a cholesterol medication known as a statin, your levels are even lower as statins will reduce CoQ10.

Supplementing with CoQ10 has been shown to reduce BP by 15–18/10 points. This is significant and can make the difference of whether medications are needed or not. If you're on BP meds and you start taking CoQ10, monitor your BP as it can lower it enough that the meds may need to be reduced.

And here's another point about CoQ10. For best absorption, it should be ubiquinone. Normal doses are between 100 and 200 mg daily.

Hawthorn. This is a flowering shrub that is part of the rose family. It has a red berry fruit that has been used for years for medicinal purposes, including lowering BP, treating congestive heart failure, decreasing cholesterol, and treating digestive and kidney problems. It dilates the arteries, is an anti-inflammatory, and has diuretic effects. Doses are between 200 and 1,500 mg a day.

Hawthorn can interfere with quite a few drugs, so don't take this if you're also taking beta blockers, calcium channel blockers, Viagra or similar drugs, or digoxin.

Celery. Four stalks of celery a day will lower the BP by around seven points. Get used to eating celery throughout the day, and use celery seed in your cooking. Buy organic celery only, as this vegetable readily concentrates pesticides from our soil.

Pycnogenol. Usually derived from pine bark, this substance has been shown to increase NO and dilate our arteries, lowering BP by seven points on average. It also works synergistically with ACE inhibitors, so if you're on one of these meds, monitor your BP closely, as you may need to cut your dose in half. Pycnogenol also helps protect us from oxidative stress and helps lower blood sugar in those with diabetes. The typical dose is 200 mg/day.

Melatonin. Most people know this as the sleep hormone, but it actually has so many other effects than just this. Melatonin is a strong antioxidant and helps to protect women from breast cancer, men from prostate cancer, and our brains from dementia. It also treats heartburn at a dose of 6 mg per night for forty nights. Taking 3 mg nightly will help keep BP even throughout the night and helps to maintain a normal circadian rhythm. Beta blockers reduce melatonin, so if you're on one of these drugs, you may need between 3 and 6 mg per night.

People always ask, What about salt? Shouldn't I restrict the amount of salt in my diet? The answer for most of us is no! Only about 10% of us are actually sensitive to salt, and those will need to reduce salt intake to less than 2,500 mg/day. How do you know if you're sensitive to salt? If you tend to get fluid retention easily, where your ankles and/or hands will swell, you may be sensitive to salt.

The best salt to use is sea salt as it is rich in minerals. Celtic or pink Himalayan sea salt are the best, with sixty to eighty-four minerals, and should be used daily.

Can these supplements really work such that you don't have to take medications for BP? Absolutely, yes. I've seen it time and time again. You don't need to take all of them, of course, but pick several and start several months before your DOT is due.

Just ask Ted, a forty-eight-year-old whose blood pressure began to increase around age forty and now is in the range requiring treatment, averaging 152/102. He knew his DOT was coming up in four months, so I had him start taking slow-release L-arginine for three tabs twice a day, 400 mg of magnesium glycinate at night, 100 mg/day of CoQ10, 5,000 IU/day of Vitamin D, 3 mg of melatonin at night, and increased his protein, decreasing carb intake. His weight dropped ten pounds in six weeks, and after two months, the BP normalized to 132/78. After another two months, the BP dropped to 126/72, and his weight was down another five pounds.

Marie was on three different meds for hypertension, and her BP was still too high. She was already restricted to yearly DOT exams, but she was facing the prospect of losing her DOT completely if her BP would not go down. Since she was a single mom and the only breadwinner of the family, this prospect caused her great anxiety.

Even with three meds, her BP was 160/98. After excluding other potential causes of hypertension, I started her on an aggressive three-month program with L-arginine, magnesium, hawthorn, vitamin D, vitamin C, CoQ10, and celery. It was lots of celery—four to five stalks daily. After three months, her BP actually dropped too low to 110/ 62, and she felt dizzy and light-headed when she stood up. She was able to eventually come off two of her meds and now is well controlled, with no danger of losing her DOT. As an added bonus, she's now more motivated to exercise and eat better and has lost twenty-four pounds so far.

What if you have limited funds and can only afford one or two? Start with magnesium and L-arginine. This will give you the biggest bang for your buck. And eat your celery and citrus!

Chapter 5

Obstructive Sleep Apnea

Worrying does not empty tomorrow of its troubles . . . it empties today of its strengths.

—Corrie ten Boom

Jason has driven a truck since age twenty, and it has enabled him a good living. He is able to provide a home for his family. But lately, his wife has been complaining that his snoring is getting louder, and at times, she's noted that he gasps at night. To get a good night's sleep, she'll often leave the room and sleep in another bedroom. He's also waking up with a headache in the morning and has noticed more fatigue or tiredness during the day.

The diagnosis of obstructive sleep apnea, or OSA, in our truck drivers is more and more common, with the newer federal regulations put in place. What is OSA?

Obstructive sleep apnea is a sleep disorder where there is a significant decrease or complete stoppage of airflow in the presence of breathing effort. It's the most common type of sleep-disordered breathing and occurs when there is recurrent upper airway collapse during sleep. It's basically a mechanical problem. During sleep, the tongue falls back against the soft palate, or roof of the mouth, and the soft palate and uvula fall back against the back of the throat, effectively closing the airway.

Breathing pauses can last from a few seconds to minutes and can occur twenty to seventy times an hour and can last at least ten seconds or more. Typically, normal breathing occurs again with a gasping, snorting, or choking sound. Since there's an abrupt airway cutoff, the oxygen decreases, and patients with OSA will have low oxygen throughout the night. It also does not allow for consistent deep sleep, which causes tiredness during the day.

Why is sleep apnea for truckers so important? Because OSA is the number 1 cause of excessive daytime sleepiness, leading to falling asleep at the wheel. Studies have shown that a third of truck drivers have mild to moderate OSA, and many are undiagnosed. A November 2014 report by the AAA Foundation for Traffic Safety estimated drowsy driving causes 328,000 crashes, 109,000 injuries, and 6,400 deaths each year. Commercial drivers are more likely to drive drowsy, according to the CDC.

The number 1 symptom of sleep apnea is snoring. Oftentimes, a spouse will hear gasping or snorting in addition to loud snoring. Other symptoms include

- excessive daytime sleepiness,
- morning headaches and/or nausea,
- foggy brain or difficulty with concentration,
- heartburn,
- irritability,
- loss of sex drive and erectile dysfunction,
- difficulty losing weight with abdominal obesity, and
- frequent nighttime urination.

Untreated sleep apnea makes it difficult to focus, stay alert, and react quickly when needed. It is indisputable that drivers with untreated sleep apnea have a higher risk of motor vehicle accidents. It may not be as obvious as falling asleep at the wheel, but the delayed reflexes leads to slow reaction times and inattentiveness, greatly increasing the risk of accidents.

Other health risks of untreated OSA are many—increased risk of a heart attack, stroke, high blood pressure, depression, atrial fibrillation, heart failure, headache, and diabetes. Having untreated sleep apnea will cut a decade or more off your life!

Up until the summer of 2017, it was required to screen for OSA with certain parameters, and if positive, then it required treatment. Now, however, the screening and treatment of OSA is *not* required, and it is now up to the individual trucking company.

Before, to be flagged that you might have OSA at the time of your DOT exam required one of two things: a neck circumference of seventeen inches for men and sixteen for women or a BMI of 35 or higher.

If you have one or both of these, you may be required to have a test to rule out sleep apnea.

Other risk factors for having OSA are age greater than sixty, enlarged tonsils, chronic nasal congestion, smoking, being male, family history, alcohol use, and high blood pressure; and some studies have suggested that African Americans have a higher risk.

While FMCSA regulations no longer specifically address sleep apnea, they do prescribe that a person with a medical history or clinical diagnosis of any condition likely to interfere with their ability to drive safely cannot be medically qualified to operate a commercial motor vehicle in interstate commerce.

If you're flagged to have testing done and if it's is required by your company, you'll be given a three-month certification to allow enough time to complete diagnostic testing and, if positive, start treatment.

The diagnosis of OSA is a sleep study. This can be done at a sleep lab, but if your town is like ours, it will take four to six months to get in, and no one can actually sleep in the lab with wires hooked to every surface of your body (or so it seems), with a camera watching your every move, and in a bed that isn't your own. You'll be billed $4,000+ for the night, which will probably be applied to your deductible, meaning you'll have to pay the whole thing. A simpler way? Home sleep studies!

A home sleep study can be ordered by your doctor or through us, and you'll be sent home with instructions on how to use it. You sleep in your own bed with minimal intervention as compared to a sleep lab. The results are very accurate, and usually, we'll have them within one week. Then based on results, treatment can be initiated if needed. Federal regulations do allow home sleep testing. But don't try to outsmart them. They have built-in computers and know if you're the one using them.

If you have a cold or nasal congestion, wait till the symptoms are gone before doing the test to increase your chances of passing.

Still afraid you might fail the test because your spouse has complained of your snoring? There are two other simple things you can do that might increase your chances of passing the test and reduce any apnea:

1. *Deep breathing.* A cause of sleep apnea can be because their breathing has become weak. The muscles of respiration can become weak when our breathing pattern is shallow and, therefore, not used properly; this can contribute to apnea. In this case, practice a simple exercise—a deep-breathing technique. Sit or lie down and take a deep breath through your

nose, watching your abdomen expand and then your lungs to a slow count of four. Hold your breath to a count of four, then let it back out through your nose to a count of six. Repeat ten times twice daily, especially right before bed. This simple exercise will slowly strengthen your breathing.

2. *Sleep apnea relief.* This is an herbal remedy that helps you breathe deeper. It's a combination of lobelia, thyme, meadowsweet, chamomile, and cramp bark in the capsule. This combination helps stimulate stronger breathing and helps avoid the stops in breathing and dangerous drops in oxygen levels at night. These stops in breathing trigger the characteristic snort of sleep apnea. It relaxes the diaphragm, the main breathing muscle, and increases drowsiness. Take one capsule at night. If you weigh over 220 pounds, take two. For most people, the snoring, sleep apnea, and weak breathing will improve within seven to ten days.

Once you complete the apnea testing, the sleep test will come back with a score called an AHI (apnea hyponea index) or, in other words, how many times per hour you quit breathing. A score of 15 or more requires treatment.

AHI   <5, no apnea
              5–14.9, mild OSA
              15–30, moderate OSA
              >30, severe OSA

It will also tell you the level of oxygen all night—how many minutes it dipped below 90 and the lowest oxygen during the night. Normally, oxygen should not drop below 95, but I routinely see it in the 70s–80s in patients with OSA. That lack of oxygen is killing brain cells and stresses the heart, potentially leading to congestive heart failure over time.

If you're diagnosed with moderate to severe sleep apnea, it will be up to your truck company if treatment is required to maintain your CDL. The standard treatment, and by far the most common, is a machine called CPAP or continuous positive airway pressure. It forces air into the airways by using small amounts of air pressure so that your airway doesn't collapse. This also prevents snoring, which is always a blessing for the spouse. (See pic.)

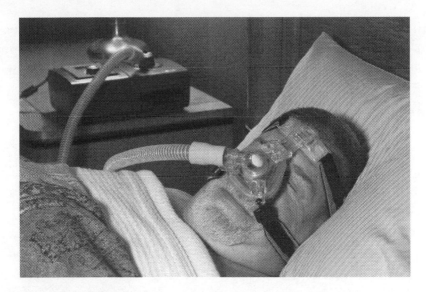

I have patients that love their CPAP and sleep soundly with it. But at least 50% of patients do not tolerate the machine and are not able to get restful sleep. The mask can be uncomfortable, or they may not be able to sleep in the position that they're used to. Some patients feel claustrophobic and tear the mask off in the middle of the night.

Another problem with the CPAP is infection. If the machine is not kept clean, it can lead to increased risk of bronchitis, pneumonia, and sinus infections. Recently, the concern is that a biofilm may be developing in the tubing of the CPAP. A biofilm is a growth of a mixture of different microbes on a surface, and they make infections much harder to treat. Many different microbes have been colonized on CPAP tubing or the filters, including MRSA (methicillin resistant staph), TB (tuberculosis), bacteria, and mold.

If you're using a CPAP, pay attention to cleaning and make sure you do this consistently. Your CPAP company will show you how. Typically, there's a daily routine and a weekly cleaning that needs to be done.

To show compliance with your CPAP so that your insurance continues to pay for it, you must wear your CPAP at least four hours a night (70% of the time). The machines have built-in computers in them and give a report on how often they're being used. This information will be relayed to your primary care physician.

Another treatment for OSA is with an oral appliance. According to the American Academy of Sleep Medicine guidelines, oral appliance therapy is indicated as a first-line therapy with mild and moderate OSA and also can be used with severe OSA when a patient has failed or refused CPAP. How does it work? With OSA, the airway is blocked by the tongue during sleep. The oral appliance keeps the lower jaw forward during sleep, which keeps the tongue forward. Side effects include TMJ pain, tooth movement, and bite changes; so seeing a dentist with the proper training is absolutely necessary.

Surgery can also be an option with OSA, but it is often not successful. If the tonsils are obviously enlarged, this may be enough. Another surgery is one called a UPPP or uvulopalatopharyngoplasty, a fancy word for an extremely painful surgery where the uvula, the tissue that hangs down in the back of the throat, is cut off along with some of the surrounding tissue.

The most effective treatment for OSA is weight loss. I had a patient that was diagnosed with severe sleep apnea in October, with an AHI of forty-seven times per hour. He hated his CPAP and, therefore, was extremely motivated to lose weight. By April, he had lost seventy pounds! We repeated his sleep study, and he no longer had the condition. We were able then to extend his DOT back to two years, with the warning that if he regains the weight, he'll be back to square one.

That being said, I do have thin patients with OSA, so it's not always a guarantee that weight loss will be the cure. However, it helps with so many other conditions, so it is always recommended.

Other alternative treatments for sleep apnea include the following:

Night shift. This is a device that is worn on the back of the neck. It vibrates when you lie on your neck, causing you to wake up enough to roll back to your side. It is effective only for patients with sleep apnea on their back but not sides. The home sleep test will tell you the AHI of both supine (on the back) or nonsupine (on the sides) and, therefore, will let you know if this would work for you. The nonsupine must be an AHI of 15 or less.

Hypoglossal nerve stimulation. This is a recent therapy that involves stimulation of the hypoglossal nerve—the nerve that controls tongue movement. An implant is placed in the body that's similar to a pacemaker, and when the hypoglossal nerve is stimulated, it moves the tongue forward to open the space for breathing. This is new enough that at this time, it often is not covered by insurance and may not meet FMCSA guidelines for treatment.

Once diagnosed with sleep apnea and proper treatment is started, you may be required to be recertified annually. Unless, of course, you can reverse it, as the patient above did. You'll also need to show compliance with the method you're using.

There is another type of sleep apnea called central sleep apnea. This type is much less common and is when the brain doesn't send proper signals to the respiratory muscles to breathe properly. It usually occurs as a result of other conditions, such as stroke, heart failure, and medications. It is treated differently than OSA, often requiring oxygen, treatment of the underlying medical problems, and a device called adaptive servo-ventilation. This technology utilizes positive airway pressure ventilator support that is adjusted based on the detection of apneas or the pauses in breathing during sleep.

Chapter 6

HEART DISEASE

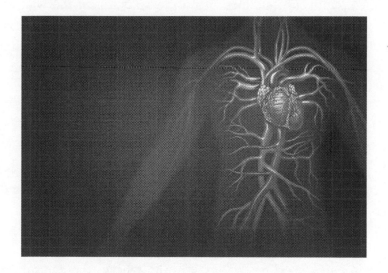

The pessimist sees difficulty in every opportunity. The optimist sees opportunity in every difficulty.

—Winston Churchill

Heart disease is the number 1 killer of all Americans. Rich or poor, male or female, black or white, it doesn't matter. It kills more than all cancers combined, yet we're always more afraid of cancer. What exactly do we mean by heart disease?

When we generally speak about heart disease, we're usually talking about coronary artery disease or CAD. This is where the arteries of the heart, called the coronary arteries, become clogged with plaque and don't allow sufficient blood flow to the heart. This narrowing of the arteries is called atherosclerosis.

If the arteries in the neck, called the carotid arteries, are narrowed, this can cause strokes as it restricts blood flow to the brain. Narrowing of the arteries to the kidney can cause high blood pressure. Narrowing of the leg arteries can cause pain in the calves when walking called claudication. We'll address this in more detail in the later chapter. Plaque buildup in the aorta, the main artery of the body in the abdomen, can cause an aneurysm or weakening of the wall of the artery. If an abdominal aortic aneurysm gets to five centimeters or larger, it is at risk of rupture, which can lead to death in two minutes. Therefore, if they are discovered, they can be repaired before this devastating event occurs.

Chest pain from CAD is called angina. And it simply means the heart muscle is starving of oxygen. Often, you'll feel the pain with exertion when you're walking or doing some other activity that requires you to breathe more. This then requires the heart to pump harder, and the heart needs more blood flow to do so but doesn't get it because the arteries are clogged.

The pain can sometimes be just a mild ache in the central or left side of the chest. Occasionally, it radiates into the left arm and/or jaw. Other times, it can be felt as an elephant sitting on the chest or a feeling of pressure.

Anytime you feel this type of pain, you must be seen urgently. And if the pain does not go away after rest or within ten minutes, go to the nearest ER. It could be an actual heart attack or MI (myocardial infarction). Other symptoms of an MI include nausea, feeling clammy, sweating, and back pain.

What are the risk factors for heart disease? Quite a few, with the most common being the following:

- *Age.* After age fifty, our risk increases yearly.
- *Male sex.* More men than women die of heart attacks, though heart disease is the number 1 cause of death in women as well as men.
- *Inflammation.* This is the biggest risk factor. Heart disease is a disease of inflammation, not a disease of cholesterol! I can't stress this enough.

You must know your inflammatory markers to adequately know your risk of CAD. Markers of inflammation include the following:

- *hs-CRP or high-sensitivity C-reactive protein.* Optimal levels are less than 1. Normal is 1–3. Anything more than 3 puts you at higher risk. The most common cause of elevated hs-CRP is abdominal obesity—fat cells around the abdomen or beer belly.
- *MPO or myeloperoxidase.* This is a marker of inflammation that can give a warning sign of plaque instability.
- *Lp-PLA$_2$.* This is a specific marker for vascular inflammation or risk of plaque rupture. People with elevated levels are at increased risk of stroke and heart attack. A high PLA is a much greater risk of sudden heart attack than cholesterol!
- *Diabetes.* Type 1 or type 2 DM greatly increases your risk of heart disease, stroke, Alzheimer's, high blood pressure, kidney failure, blindness, cancer, and peripheral artery disease or plaque buildup in the leg arteries. Why? Because DM greatly increases *inflammation* that is the cause of all chronic disease.
- *Smoking.* This highly addictive habit greatly increases inflammation and causes spasms of the coronary arteries, leading to sudden heart attacks.

- *Family history of early heart disease before age sixty.* This can potentially increase your risk as well.
- *Obesity.* Being overweight or obese increases inflammation, which, as stated above, increases risk of heart attacks and strokes.
- *Low testosterone in men.* Replacing testosterone as men age will reduce the risk of heart disease, and this will be discussed in more detail in chapter.
- *Menopause in women.* After women go through menopause, their risk of heart disease begins to increase to equal men's, unless they start hormone replacement. This will be discussed further in chapter.

But what about cholesterol? Isn't that a major risk factor of heart disease, if not the number 1 risk factor? No! We need to learn the truth about cholesterol and why it is a minimal, if at all, risk factor for coronary artery disease. The truth is that a high cholesterol is found in only 50% of all heart attacks. The other half has low levels, with a third of patients below 160.

Cholesterol is critical for our health. It is a waxy, fat-like substance found in every cell membrane and is needed for many different functions:

- It makes our hormones, especially the sex hormones—testosterone and estrogen.
- We need cholesterol in our skin to activate vitamin D3 for sunlight.
- It is necessary for brain health, as 25% of the brain is cholesterol. When levels are driven too low, as with statin drugs, memory loss can occur.
- It plays a big role in helping fight bacteria and infections. A study that included one hundred thousand healthy people over fifteen years found that those with low cholesterol were

much more likely to be admitted to hospitals with infectious diseases.

The worst thing that was done for the health of our society was to replace saturated fats with carbohydrates, which has greatly increased the risk for heart disease. This has contributed to the increase in heart disease we've seen in the last twenty-plus years.

The fact is that lowering cholesterol has a very limited benefit in populations other than middle-aged men who've already had a heart attack or those who have a coronary stent or bypass surgery. Statin drugs—which include Lipitor (atorvastatin), Zocor (simvastatin), Crestor (rosuvastatin), Pravachol (pravastatin), and Lescol (fluvastatin)—are the most commonly used drugs to lower cholesterol. And they are widely overprescribed.

One example of this was shown with a drug called Vytorin. This was a combination cholesterol-lowering drug that the drug company Merck had invested tremendous amount of money in making. This new *wonder* drug lowered cholesterol better than any standard statin drug. So lower the cholesterol then lower the heart disease, right?

No, not quite. Although it did cause cholesterol levels to plummet, the patients actually had *more* plaque growth, with an almost twice as great an increase in the thickness of their arterial walls.

There are countless other studies with similar findings, but another one worth mentioning is one called the Nurses' Health Study. Conducted by Harvard University, this is one of the longest-running studies of diet and disease ever done. The study has followed more than 120,000 females since the mid-1970s to determine risk factors for cancer and heart disease. In the final analysis, as published in the *New England Journal of Medicine*, five factors were identified that significantly lowered the risk of heart disease. They are the following: don't smoke, drink alcohol only in moderation, engage in moderate to vigorous exercise for at least half an hour a day, keep BMI less than 25, and eat a wholesome, low-sugar diet with plenty of omega-3 fats and fiber. Cholesterol had absolutely nothing to do with it!

Why isn't this more publicized? The inconvenient truth that lowering cholesterol has almost no effect on extending life is ignored by the special interests that profit enormously from keeping this information from you, the consumer. Statins produce $30 billion a year in gross revenue, and the drug companies, or Big Pharma, have tremendous power in our country and over the FDA.

Another study worth mentioning is one done in 1991 by two doctors who published a book called *The Cholesterol Conspiracy*. They reviewed all the cholesterol-lowering trials that had been done up to that time. They found that the drugs work great at lowering cholesterol but nothing else. In the vast majority of the studies reviewed, there was no difference in the death rate for those on statin drugs and those who weren't. And in some cases, more people died who were on the drugs.

There is one good thing about statin drugs, however. They lower inflammation, which, as we know, is the cause of all chronic disease. This is the reason why, in some cases, they can provide some benefit. But the dose to do that is very low. I've prescribed a drug like Crestor at 5 mg for three times a week to someone with known plaque buildup.

What are the problems with statin drugs? There are many, including the following:

- They deplete CoQ10, a vital nutrient needed in the heart, brain, and muscle cells. Anyone on a statin drug should take CoQ10, at least 100–200 mg/day. Depletion of CoQ10 can cause muscle weakness, fatigue, and foggy brain.

- They lead to a reduction in sex hor+mones. Cholesterol is the building block of all our hormones, and when levels get too low, especially under 150, testosterone and estrogen are reduced. Sexual dysfunction is a common side effect, and in men, statins are often associated with ED or erectile dysfunction.
- They increase the risk of dementia. The brain depends heavily on cholesterol to function well, and it contains 25% of the body's cholesterol. Memory loss commonly occurs with these drugs, and they can be devastating in the elderly for this reason. Statins should never be used past age eighty! Even transient global amnesia has occurred with these drugs, which is not always reversible.
- They double the risk of diabetes in women. And we know that diabetes greatly increases inflammation, heart disease, and kidney disease.
- They increase the risk of neuropathy or nerve pain. I'll never forget a fifty-four-year-old male patient of mine with extremely painful nerve pain in both arms. After extensive workup, it was found that his pain was due to Lipitor. Unfortunately, even after stopping the drug, he had suffered permanent damage, with some wasting of the muscles in the upper arm and continuous nerve pain.
- They change the neurotransmitters in the brain and can cause depression or cause antidepressants to not be as effective.
- There are studies showing that the risk of cancer is significantly associated with lower LDL cholesterol levels.

But if all this is true, then why, in the media, do we always hear that statins reduce heart disease by 20–30%? Because of fuzzy math. Studies will tout that their drug lowers cholesterol by 28% but will not tell you that there was no reduction in heart attacks. Or as seen in the heart protection study, look at patients on Zocor versus those on placebo. Those on Zocor had an 87.1% survival rate after five years, while those on placebo had an 85.4% survival rate. This is an absolute difference of 1.8%. And the survival rates were independent of lowering cholesterol. But the study claimed *massive benefits* by lowering cholesterol with a statin drug.

I could give example after example, and for those of you who want to know more, I urge you read the book *The Great Cholesterol Myth* by Dr. Stephen Sinatra, a well-respected cardiologist who also practices antiaging medicine.

We also know that patients who live into their nineties have an average cholesterol of 225. This seems to be a healthy number for the body and brain as we age.

So the bottom line is that cholesterol is a very minor factor, if any at all, for heart disease. Much more important is inflammation, lifestyle, healthy weight, diet, and exercise.

We'll have a word about fats, and we'll get into this more on the nutrition chapter. There are good fats and bad fats, and the bad fats need to be avoided like poison, which they are. Bad fats include the following:

- *Trans fats.* For each 2% increase in trans fat calories consumed, the risk for heart disease *doubles*. The worst offenders are nondairy creamers, which are actually just chemicals; margarine, which is one molecule away from plastic; soup cups; ramen noodles; fast food; all packaged baked goods like Twinkies and crackers; donuts; cereals; and many energy bars.
- *Omega-6 fats.* Vegetable oils—such as canola, corn, soybean, and safflower—are highly inflammatory. They are hard to avoid, as nearly all processed food has them. Do not have them in your kitchen!

- *Marg*arine. This is a yellow chemical spread made to look like butter and is inflammatory. Use butter. Never, ever use margarine.

The good oils that reduce inflammation and help with brain and heart function include the following:

- Omega-3 (at a dose of 3,000–4,000 mg a day for most of us).
- Avocado oil.
- Coconut oil.
- Nut and seed oil.
- Olive oil (but it must be dark, extra-virgin, and in a glass bottle). The cheap light olive oil in plastic has been bleached to make it light, and the plastic causes oxidation, ruining the oil.
- Grape-seed oil.

There are important nutrients and foods for the heart, chief among them are the following:

- *Omega-3s.* These are extremely important to reduce the risk of heart disease and stroke, and they also reduce asthma flares and help keep joints supple. Take between 3,000 and 4,000 mg/day (divide in two doses). Take with food, and make sure that your brand is mercury and toxin free. It should say it on the label. Wild salmon is also a good source of omega-3, but avoid farm-raised salmon, which are lower in omega-3, and are contaminated with PCBs and other toxins.
- *CoQ10.* Must be taken in 100–200 mg/day doses, preferably in ubiquinone form. This is vital for the heart and brain. Take with vitamin E. This lowers CRP, or C-reactive protein, even lower.
- *Pomegranate juice.* One-fourth cup a day helps to keep the arteries flexible and reduces plaque buildup by 30% more than any drug! It also enhances the activity of nitric oxide.

- *Cherries, raspberries, and blackberries.* These have a high amount of anthocyanins for reducing inflammation.
- *D-Ribose.* This is essential for energy production. I use it in those with congestive heart failure or chronic fatigue, at a dose of 5 g two to three times a day for those with heart disease and up to 20 g daily for those with advanced heart disease or frequent angina.
- *Acetyl-L-Carnitine.* Studies have shown that those taking L-carnitine after heart attacks had significantly lower mortality rates. They took them at a dose of 2 g daily. It improves blood flow to the limbs and to the heart and can reduce episodes of angina.
- *Magnesium.* This is essential for so many functions, and most of us are low in this nutrient. Lower levels increase risk of heart disease. Supplement with at least 400 mg a day. Magnesium oxide is the cheapest form and is not well absorbed, instead causing diarrhea. Take either magnesium glycinate, citrate, or chelate.
- *Vitamin E.* This is a strong antioxidant. It also helps to increase blood flow to the heart. Most E sold is the cheap alpha-tocopherol. To be effective, the E must be a combination of eight related compounds: four tocopherols and four tocotrienols in the form of alpha, delta, beta, and gamma. Take 200 IU daily.
- *Resveratrol.* This is known for its antiaging activity. It helps protect the arteries by making them more flexible, lowering blood pressure, inhibiting blood clots, and lowering oxidized LDL. Take 20–200 mg of trans-resveratrol—the active component and the only kind that works.
- *B complex.* This is needed for energy production in the heart, brain, and muscles.
- *Vitamin C.* The lower the level of this vitamin, the higher the risk for heart failure and atherosclerosis. Eat foods with C every day, such as fruits and vegetables, and take between

1,000 and 4,000 mg a day. If it starts to cause diarrhea, back off.

You'll notice I didn't include aspirin. For most of us, aspirin is not needed as long as we take our fish oil. Aspirin taken long-term can increase risk of macular degeneration (a form of blindness), kidney disease, and stomach ulcers.

The worst foods for the heart are the trans fats, sugar, processed carbohydrates, soda, processed meat, and excessive omega-6 fats. All these increase inflammation and atherosclerosis or plaque buildup. As you get rid of these in your diet, you'll find that a nice side effect will occur—weight loss.

If you have heart disease, there is much you can do to repair and even reverse the damage. Be proactive and start with small simple things one step at a time, and your heart will thank you!

Chapter 7

GERD—Heartburn

You don't have to have it all figured out to move forward.

Heartburn—otherwise known as GERD or gastroesophageal reflux disease—is a common complaint in our society. At one time or another, almost all of us have felt the burn of acid coming from our stomach and into our esophagus. Symptoms are typically a burning sensation in our midchest, and it can rise all the way up to our throat. Sometimes it's felt only in our throat or may cause a chronic sore throat. When the ear/nose/throat doctors take a look, they can see the red and swollen vocal cords.

Other symptoms of GERD include a chronic cough, and if you have asthma, it can cause a worsening of your asthma with increased need to use your inhaler. While not affecting a DOT exam, the symptoms of GERD can make life miserable.

Ted first noticed heartburn after eating, and he would drink an antacid to put out the fire. Eventually, this stopped working, and he started taking over-the-counter Prilosec or the generic, omeprazole. Soon he had to take a pill every day, sometimes twice a day. But who cared? What did it really matter, as long as the pill worked, and he wasn't having any more symptoms of burning in his throat?

GERD is caused by incomplete closure of the sphincter between the esophagus and stomach, allowing the stomach acid to come up and irritate the lining of the esophagus and throat.

Anything that increases the pressure in the abdomen can cause GERD, such as pregnancy, abdominal fat, or simply eating too big a meal like we do at Thanksgiving or the greasy foods often eaten in a hurry at the local truck stop. But these episodes are usually short-lived and can be easily treated with some baking soda, lemon water, or apple cider vinegar.

For Americans, 40% suffer from heartburn every month, and it's the chronic GERD that's the problem. If chronic acid exposure on the tissue of the esophagus is not treated, this can lead to abnormal cells that can potentially turn into cancer of the esophagus. So it does need to be addressed.

However, the drugs that are used to treat GERD are widely misused. Drugs such as Prilosec, Protonix, Nexium, Prevacid, AcipHex, or Zegerid were originally made to be used for only two weeks. Of course, this isn't done, and instead, they are being used indefinitely for years. Now they generate more than $14 billion a year for the drug companies.

What is the impact of taking a drug that blocks the stomach-acid production? Many. The acidic environment of the stomach is needed for many reasons, including proper digestion and absorption of nutrients. Because of this, the drugs are associated with many risks, including

- increased risk of dementia;
- osteoporosis;
- increased risk of stroke and heart disease by decreasing nitric oxide;
- more infections with *C. difficile* and pneumonia;
- protein deficiency; and
- deficiency of B12, magnesium, calcium, and iron.

What causes GERD? Conventionally, it's taught that GERD is caused by too much stomach acid or HCl, but this is simply not true. Rather, GERD is caused by too *little* stomach acid! Let's look at a picture of the stomach. Imagine a constantly moving, rolling pouch filled up with hydrochloric acid with a pH of 1 and enzymes that are churning to break down protein and other food that is delivered to the sack. The stomach lining secretes a thick mucus that coats the lining to protect it from the acid. If it weren't there, the stomach would be digested by the acid it secretes.

But with GERD, there is often too little stomach acid, and because of this, the food, especially protein, cannot be broken down and digested well, leading to belching and bad breath. Also, the sphincter is stimulated to shut tightly when there is acid. When there isn't enough HCl acid, your sphincter may relax and allow the stomach contents to come up.

After a heavy meal, the pressure in the stomach can increase so much that the sphincter can open, allowing the bile and acid back up into the esophagus, with the all-too-familiar burn felt in our chest. Belching and a sour taste in the mouth can also occur.

So if the meds for heartburn are bad for us long-term, how do we treat the condition? We've got to get to the root of the disease and fix the problem. Natural treatments for heartburn include the following:

- First of all, since most people with heartburn have too little stomach acid, we need to give some acid back. The easiest way is to take something called betaine with digestive enzymes. Take one at the beginning of a meal and one midway during the meal. The more protein you're eating, the more acid you need.
- Another way of getting HCl is with apple cider vinegar. Take one tablespoon of raw, unfiltered apple cider vinegar, and mix it with eight ounces of water and drink before each meal,

three times a day. If you try this for two days and it worsens your reflux, then stop. You might be one of those who has enough HCl.

- Chew a piece of sugar-free gum for one half hour after your meal. This encourages the saliva to flow and dilutes the acid in the gut, washing it back down.
- Drink lemon water throughout the day. It's best to use a fresh lemon, squeezing the juice of the lemon in a liter of water and drinking it during the day. Use lemon essential oil in your water. It works great too.
- Eat okra. If you've ever eaten okra, you're from the south and know that this is a slimy food. The slime coats the stomach and helps it to heal.
- Don't lie down within three to four hours after eating. Lying down with a full stomach puts too much pressure on that sphincter, allowing stomach contents to come up.
- Take 6 mg of melatonin at night, once a night, for forty nights. There are melatonin receptors in the esophagus and stomach, and it helps these tissues to heal.
- Zinc carnosine is also very effective at completely healing GERD. Take 75 mg a day for one month.
- Eat mustard. This spice is a food that contains many minerals and contains a weak acid. If you feel heartburn coming up, take one teaspoon of straight mustard.
- Maintain a healthy weight and make sure your pants aren't too tight. Extra pounds will put pressure on the sphincter, causing it to weaken.
- Don't smoke or drink. Both alcohol and nicotine relaxes the sphincter, allowing acid reflux to occur more easily.
- Eat three to four almonds after every meal. They help to neutralize some of the digestive juices in the stomach.
- Probiotics can help you have a healthy intestinal tract, and I recommend taking one every day. They need to have at least eight strains of probiotics and at least ten billion per capsule.

After age fifty, most of us don't make enough HCl and need to start supplementing in combination with digestive enzymes with our meals.

I use a ninety-day program to get people off PPIs. Start betaine and digestive enzymes with meals (6 mg of melatonin at night, 75 mg of zinc carnosine for one month), drink lemon water with lemon essential oil, chew gum, eat almonds, and avoid eating before bed. After two weeks, we'll stop the PPI then start 150 mg/day of Zantac. (You can get this over the counter.) Take the Zantac for two weeks, then stop. Expect an increase in heartburn for three days, as your stomach is happy that it finally gets to make acid again. Keep drinking your lemon water and apple cider vinegar and taking the supplements, and 85% of the time, you will be permanently off these drugs. For the 15% that fail, it is safer to be on a drug like Zantac or Tagamet rather than a PPI, and as you lose weight, the heartburn will continue to improve.

Remember, a healthy gut is a healthy body!

Chapter 8

DEEP VENOUS THROMBOSIS— BLOOD CLOTS

It always seems impossible until it is done.

—Nelson Mandela

Matt is a long-haul truck driver. He was halfway across the country when he woke up one morning and noticed some swelling of his leg and a little tenderness when he put his weight on it. Thinking he might have sprained it, he got back in the truck to start his eleven-hour day. Then several hours later, he noticed a pain in his right chest that was rather sharp and a cough. His next thought was that he was getting sick, a respiratory infection of some kind probably. When he made a stop to refuel and for a bathroom break, he finally started to get worried when he noticed he was short of breath after just walking and doing minimal exertion. Now the pain was worse, sharp and searing, and what finally made him drive to the nearest ER was when he coughed up blood. Testing revealed a large blood clot in his left leg that extended from calf to thigh and a pulmonary embolism, or blood clot, in his right lung. He was hospitalized for three days then was sent home on blood thinners—initially Lovenox shots, then Coumadin.

There are hazards to sitting for long periods. And one that unfortunately is all too common is DVT or deep venous thrombosis. It's basically a blood clot in the deep veins of the legs. Those that sit for four or more hours have a 48% higher risk of mortality from DVT. For those with DVT, 30% will die within one month; 25% of these will occur as sudden death! The recurrence rate is 33% within ten years. And up to one hundred thousand Americans die every year from blood clots. Of course, this also includes clots as a complication of surgery or in the postoperative period.

There are both superficial veins and deep veins in our extremities. The superficial veins can be seen as a bluish coloration of the veins, and sometimes varicose veins develop. These varicose veins may be unsightly, but they are not dangerous. Occasionally, they can get inflamed, red and sore, but they are not life-threatening.

Deep veins are not visible, but they are deep in the arms and legs. A DVT can form in the legs, typically in the calf or thigh. The most common scenario is waking up with pain in the calf and swelling. Usually, it's just one leg, not both, and it will hurt to walk or squeeze your calf. (See pic.)

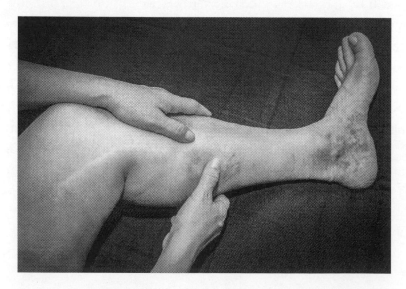

While a blood clot can form anywhere in the body, the most common is in the leg from prolonged sitting. The sitting and inactivity can cause the blood flow to be sluggish, causing clots to form. Other risk factors besides prolonged sitting include smoking, obesity, and in women, taking birth control pills. If there's a family history of clotting, you could have a genetic predisposition, and this is easy to check with a blood test called factor V Leiden.

DVTs can permanently damage the veins, causing swelling that never completely goes away. But the real damage of a DVT is if a piece breaks off, goes upstream, and lodges in the lung. This causes sharp chest pain and shortness of breath, and if the clot is large enough, it can cause death.

This is not as uncommon as you might think. If you do develop a blood clot, you'll be disqualified for at least three months and need to show that you're stable on a blood thinner for at least a month. You'll also need to be able to stop and walk every two to three hours to keep your blood circulating to help prevent another clot.

Other things you can do to help prevent a DVT is calf exercises. Simply move your feet up and down to make your calves contract. When you stop for any reason, walk at least twice around your truck.

There are supplements you can take to keep the blood flowing and reduce your risk of DVT. These include the following:

- Take 2,000 mg of fish oil twice a day with food. This must be a pure mercury-free fish oil, and you shouldn't be burping it up. It helps to keep the platelets from sticking and may enhance the breakup of clots.
- Hawthorn with grape-seed extract supports blood vessel function.
- L-arginine increases nitric oxide and improves blood flow and circulation.

- Vitamin E improves platelet flow and blood flow. In a 2007 study in the journal *Circulation*, vitamin E supplementation may reduce the risk of venous clots, and those with a prior history or genetic predisposition may particularly benefit. Eat vitamin E–rich foods like walnuts, almonds, sunflower seeds, hazelnuts, broccoli, avocado, spinach, and olive oil.
- Garlic keeps platelets from being sticky.
- Nattokinase is a natural blood thinner derived from a Japanese food called natto. It helps support the body in breaking up unhealthy coagulation of blood.
- Drink tea that's green and/or black. This contains salicylates to keep the blood flowing. Pineapple juice also does this.
- Drink ginger tea or eat ginger slices. Add fresh and dried ginger to your cooking. It helps thin the blood and improves circulation in the arteries and veins.
- Cayenne pepper is a natural blood thinner and improves circulation. Use it in your cooking, and you can take one in a capsule.
- Apple cider vinegar works great for many things, especially blood flow and circulation. It will help reduce clotting, and if you have a clot, it helps reduce pain and swelling. Add one to two tablespoons of raw, unfiltered apple cider vinegar to a glass of water, and add a little honey for taste. Drink twice daily.

Pick and choose a few of these options as part of your healthy lifestyle change, and you'll be preventing the blood clots from ever occurring in the first place. But remember this activity—walk, walk, walk at every stop and move your legs to keep the blood flowing.

Chapter 9

SMOKING

Defeat is not the worst of failures. Not to have tried is the true failure.

Carla started smoking at age fifteen when it was cool. Her habit really didn't develop until age nineteen when she was smoking a half pack a day consistently. At age twenty-two, she decided to see the country and started a career as an OTR trucker. The long hours on the road led to boredom, which led to an increase in her habit. By age twenty-four, she was up to one pack per day. It seemed like everyone in her profession did the same thing, and she didn't think much of it. But she did notice the increasing cost of her habit. Every state kept increasing the taxes on a pack of cigarettes, and now a pack cost anywhere from $4.52 in North Dakota to $10.44 in New York! And this was her cost each and every day, seven days a week. By age thirty-one, she felt herself being more winded than she used to be, with a nagging cough in the morning. Her clothes all smelled like smoke. She was getting married soon and knew that they both wanted kids. She knew she had to quit and desperately tried many ways, including cold turkey, nicotine patch, nicotine gum, and then a prescription by her doctor for Chantix. Nothing had worked so far, and she was growing increasingly frustrated.

More than twice as many truck drivers smoke as the general population—51% versus 19%. This is staggering! Why do so many truckers smoke?

Once reason, of course, is boredom. Another is stress. They've picked up the habit when younger, and with the stress of being away from family and with the isolation of being in the truck, they find that smoking helps to take the edge off.

Whatever the cause, smoking in our drivers is the number 1 cause of chronic illness and mortality, more than obesity, inactivity, and a junk food diet.

The health effects of smoking are well-known, and there are a multitude of studies to back them up. They include increased risk of heart disease, lung cancer, head and neck cancer, stroke, ulcers of the stomach and esophagus, increased wrinkling of the skin, yellow discoloration of fingertips, higher risk of gum disease, reduced smell and taste, higher risk of blindness, increased risk of blood cancer, erectile dysfunction, earlier menopause in women, COPD or chronic obstructive pulmonary disease, and increased risk of infections, just to name a few.

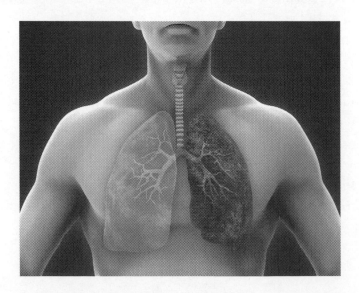

Basically, smoking harms every organ of the body and causes more than a half a million deaths in the US per year or, in other words, one in five people. If no one smoked, one in three cancer deaths wouldn't occur.

Smoking damages the lining of blood vessels, causing more plaque buildup, which causes the heart attacks, strokes, and peripheral artery disease or narrowing of the arteries in the legs.

So we know the numerous deleterious health effects of smoking and want to stop, but how? The tobacco companies knew what they were doing when they added nicotine—a highly addictive substance that enters your brain within ten seconds of taking your first puff or putting the chew in your mouth. It causes the brain to release adrenaline, which makes you feel good and energized. This buzz fades quickly, however, leaving you feeling somewhat drained and causing you to crave another cigarette to get the rush back, which creates the pattern of addiction. Nicotine is as addictive as heroin, cocaine, and methamphetamine.

Tolerance to nicotine develops quickly, which accounts for, at first, using only one to two cigarettes a day, and before you know it, you're up to one to two packs per day.

What about chewing tobacco? Isn't it safer? No! Chewing tobacco contains more nicotine than cigarettes, and putting a little in your mouth for thirty minutes is equivalent to smoking three cigarettes. Two cans of snuff a week is the same as smoking 1½ packs a day! It comes with a much higher risk of head and neck cancers.

So how do you quit the habit?

First and foremost, you must truly have the desire to quit. If you're trying to quit only because your wife is nagging you or because the doctor said to do it or you'll die, you will not succeed. This is an addiction, and any addiction is not easy to conquer. Not easy, but not impossible. You must really, really, really want this; and if you're truly motivated, you can quit smoking just as millions have already done.

Methods to quit smoking include the following:

Cold turkey. This the hardest method ever. You simply say, "I'm not going to pick up another cigarette past this date," and do it. You will start going through withdrawal within two to three hours, and symptoms include anxiety, irritability, increased hunger, headache, restlessness, and insomnia. Symptoms start to recede after a few days to a week. Then the real challenge becomes to continue to refrain from smoking, including beating the psychological addiction of hand to mouth or, in other words, the sensation of having something in your mouth or between your fingers. Oftentimes, you'll develop the tendency to chew or bite, including things like toothpicks, pretzel sticks, gum, and pens and pencils. This is one of the reasons people tend to gain weight after quitting smoking, as more and more go into the mouth.

Instead of fattening foods and carbs, choose healthier foods, such as carrot sticks, celery, sunflower seeds (the shelled ones), cinnamon or peppermint sticks, sugarless gum, and sugarless candy. Eat grapefruits—half of grapefruit four times a day. Grapefruits make cigarettes taste bad and help you detoxify.

Know your triggers and avoid them, especially during the first three months when you're more likely to relapse. And especially avoid bars and other places where there is a lot of smoke. The success rate for cold turkey is between 3% and 5%.

Nicotine patch. These are now available over the counter and come in three strengths: 21 mg, 14 mg, and 7 mg. If you smoke more than ten cigs a day, which is half a pack, then you'll use the 21 mg for six weeks, 14 mg for two weeks, and 7 mg for two weeks. You change them daily and apply to nonhairy areas of the skin. It delivers nicotine in the bloodstream to ease the withdrawal symptoms you'll experience and doubles the chances you'll be successful in beating the habit.

Nicotine gum. When you chew nicotine gum, it releases nicotine with each chew. The faster and harder you chew, the more nicotine you get. The problem is that the gum is also highly addictive, and I've known patients that have been chewing the gum for years.

Their main side effect is that the gum can completely ruin your teeth and cause severe gingivitis. Dentists can always tell when someone's been chewing nicotine gum. Other side effects include nausea, heartburn, gas, sore throat, cough, increased blood pressure, insomnia, and nightmares.

Medications (including Chantix and Wellbutrin). Chantix works by interfering with nicotine brain receptors. By doing so, it reduces symptoms of withdrawal and decreases the pleasure of cigarettes. Most people will need to take it for twelve weeks. Side effects are numerous, with the most dangerous being increased risk of suicide. I actually had this happen to a patient of mine—a young man in his thirties, who abruptly committed suicide after three weeks on this drug. It was tragic and one I will never forget, and because of this, I've been much less likely to prescribe this drug.

Other side effects of Chantix include nausea, insomnia, restlessness, changes in taste, hostility, aggressiveness, headache, and depression. There are now black box warnings for Chantix, and the drug company Pfizer has spent millions in settling lawsuits.

Wellbutrin, or bupropion, has been used longer than Chantix and is slightly less effective. You'll need to use this for twelve weeks as

well, and side effects are similar, though with a lower suicide risk than Chantix.

Do these drugs work? Chantix is reported to have a 44% success rate at twelve weeks, though this drops to 24% by six months. This compares to 23% with the patch. After one year, the success rate is 21%. Wellbutrin has similar success rates.

Electronic cigarettes. This is the newest fad, designed to give you the experience similar to smoking but without the smoke. They are touted as being safer with less cancer-causing additives and contaminants than regular cigarettes. But they are not completely safe. They still have cancer-causing contaminants and have been shown to reduce lung and heart function and to increase inflammation. There have been some explosions of the e-cigarettes while in a person's mouth, causing extensive damage.

The success rate of e-cigs has been reported to be 18% at six months. Then the difficulty is tapering the e-cigs so that this doesn't become the next expensive addiction.

Hypnosis. There is little evidence that this is effective for smokers, but like many things in alternative medicine, it does work for some. There are some studies showing that hypnosis with nicotine patches work synergistically together and increase the chances of success.

Exercise. Five minutes of intense exercise will lead to a short-term reduction in cravings, though this is hard to do when driving!

Lime juice. This will decrease cravings and has an added bonus of having significant antimicrobial properties.

Grapefruit juice. When quitting smoking, you want to flush the nicotine out of your system as quickly as possible. To do this, drink grapefruit juice. Drink a glass with each meal and in between meals. After seven days, most of the nicotine will be flushed out of your system, and this will decrease your cravings. At the same time, take 1,000 mg of vitamin C three to four times a day to help detoxify and flush out the nicotine. Diarrhea is the main side effect with C, so cut back if this occurs. Some people only tolerate 250 mg at a time.

Avoid caffeine, red meat, and alcohol. Do this as much as possible during this time. These all make cigarettes taste better.

Milk. There are a number of studies showing that milk makes cigarettes taste terrible. Drink a glass of milk whenever you are tempted to smoke and dip your cigarettes in milk and let them dry. They will taste bad enough that you may not want them anymore.

Avoid sweets. They often make you crave cigarettes.

Whatever way works for you, it is worth it to try and try again to quit smoking. When you do quit, you'll see these benefits right away:

- Within twenty minutes, your heart rate and blood pressure will drop.
- After two hours, your blood flow will increase, and the tips of your fingers will be warmer.
- Twelve hours after quitting, your carbon monoxide levels will drop, increasing your oxygen capacity.
- After one day, your risk of heart attacks will be reduced.
- Within forty-eight hours, the smell and taste nerve endings will start to regrow, and food will taste better.
- Within three weeks, your lung function will improve.
- Within nine months, your lung capacity will increase and the shortness of breath will be reduced or resolved.
- Within one year, heart disease risk will drop by half.
- Within five years, cancer risks will be reduced by half.

- After five to ten years, your risk of stroke will drop to that of a nonsmoker.
- Fifteen years later, your risk of heart disease will drop to that of a nonsmoker.

All good reasons indeed to stop this deadly habit!

Chapter 10

Depression

The past should be the past. It can destroy the future. Live life for what tomorrow has to offer, not for what yesterday has taken away.

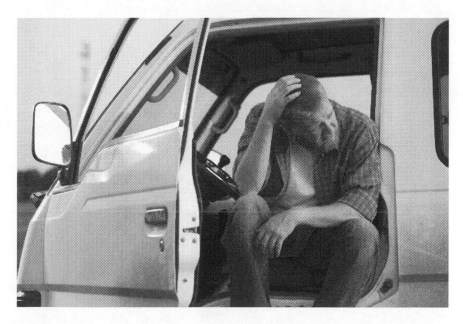

Depression is the most common mental condition that exists worldwide, affecting 350 million people and 20 million Americans. Most of us have known someone affected by this terrible condition or have ourselves been faced with the diagnosis. Yet half of those with the disorder have not been diagnosed and are, therefore, not receiving treatment, which is unfortunate since it is such a treatable disease.

What is depression? It is defined as a low mood or apathy that lasts at least two consecutive weeks and is severe enough to interrupt daily activities, including sleeping, eating, and working. It affects women more than men, at 25% versus 10%, and affects one in twenty teenagers.

Debbie drives for a small company with local deliveries in the food service industry and gets to know her customers personally. She's always enjoyed the job and the hours from 4:00 AM to noon, allowing her to be home for the kids when they get out of school. She's been married for twelve years, and her husband is supportive and helps out with the housework and with the care of their three children. Life is good with the normal stressors that are expected, and she can't understand this feeling of melancholy—a sadness that seems to permeate through her very core and a black cloud over her head. When she gets home at noon, she now wants to sleep instead of busying herself with the housework and getting dinner on the table. Meals are becoming very simple, such as macaroni and cheese and a can of olives, and she longs to climb into bed by six. She's lost interest in catching up with friends on the weekend and does not want to go out with her husband or to her kids' games and activities. She prefers to stay in bed all weekend if she could. Her family is getting stressed out that "Mom isn't the same anymore" and doesn't know how to fix the problem. She's ashamed of herself and does not want to go to the doctor and admit she has a problem.

As a physician, I see this kind of thing every day. Depression is so common in our society, and it hits every walk of life—rich or poor, young or old, male or female. Men are much more likely to turn to alcohol instead of admitting a problem, and the most common cause of alcoholism is depression.

A two-question screening tool for depression is the following:

1. Little interest or pleasure in doing things
   a. not at all
   b. several days
   c. more than half the days
   d. nearly every day

2. Feeling down, depressed, or hopeless
   a. not at all
   b. several days
   c. more than half the days
   d. nearly every day

If you answer *c* or *d* to either question, you must consider that you are suffering from depression and should seek help.

Another way to assess depression is known as SIGECAPS (sleep, interest, guilt, energy, concentration, appetite, psychomotor, and suicide). If four or more of these items are affected, it strongly suggests major depression and should be evaluated further.

Most doctors will want to start a medication, most likely something called an SSRI or selective serotonin reuptake inhibitor. These meds include Prozac, Paxil, Celexa, Lexapro, or Zoloft. Other meds used are SNRIs or serotonin norepinephrine reuptake inhibitors. These include Cymbalta, Effexor, Pristiq, and Fetzima. They block or delay the reuptake of serotonin and norepinephrine, increasing their concentration and, thereby, elevating mood.

All these drugs can be used to treat anxiety, depression, OCD (obsessive-compulsive disorder), chronic pain, and panic disorder.

Can you drive and take these meds? Yes, as long as they do not cause too much sedation. For most patients, the meds don't cause sedation, but everyone's chemistry is different. So of course, you need to see what kind of effect they will have on you. If it does make you sleepy, take it at night, which works fine as long as you're not groggy in the morning. If they tend to keep you up or cause insomnia, take them in the morning.

Common side effects include nausea (which usually goes away after one week), tiredness, restlessness, agitation, memory loss, headache, blurred vision, impotence, difficulty achieving orgasm, seizures, constipation, dry mouth, dizziness, weight loss, weight gain, increased sweating, anxiety, increased heart rate, increased blood pressure, palpitations, difficulty urinating, rash, and changes in appetite. Other more serious side effects include the following:

- The risk of suicide is doubled, especially higher in the first two months of taking it. Th
- Your risk of diabetes is two to three times higher if you take an antidepressant. The risk is so high that they now have to have a black box warning.
- The risk of a stroke may be 45% higher, related to the effect on clotting.
- There's a risk of osteoporosis or brittle bones. They are associated with a higher spinal fracture risk and 20% greater risk of all fractures;
- There's an increased risk of heart disease.
- There is a 30% higher death rate from all causes with patients taking antidepressants.

Do these drugs work? They are one of the most highly prescribed drugs, bringing in billions for the drug companies or Big Pharma. So they must work great, right? Well, not that great, and often, not at all. Numerous studies have shown that SSRIs have little benefit in those with mild to moderate depression, working no better than a placebo. And in some cases, they actually worsen depression, anxiety, and agitation, increasing the risk for violent thoughts and behaviors.

The truth is, antidepressants are *highly dangerous* and work as well as a placebo, with numerous side effects. Many of them are potentially dangerous and life-threatening. There have been numerous lawsuits against the drug companies, costing them millions. That being said, if you're on one of these drugs, you simply cannot just stop them! They must be slowly tapered, and it can be very difficult to do. I have some patients that can come off them in one month, and others have taken six months.

And if you're pregnant, talk to your doctor about getting off an SSRI or SNRI if at all possible. Studies are showing a strong correlation between these meds and autism. In other words, if you're taking the drug while pregnant, your baby has double the risk of autism. SSRIs are also associated with birth defects, such as heart defects, persistent pulmonary hypertension (a serious condition of the heart and arteries of the lungs), miscarriage, limb malformation, low birth weight, and neurological defects, including anencephaly (being born without a brain).

Whenever I have a patient with depression, I always ask the most important question, What is the root of the problem, and can it be repaired so that drugs are not needed? The answer, the vast majority of the time, is that a drug is not the answer. We can help the patient get back to feeling the excitement and joy that life has to offer using a combination of supplements and alternative treatments.

The most important thing to look at is diet. There is vast evidence that certain foods contribute to depression, and these are primarily sugar and grains. *Sugar is as addictive as heroin.* It also causes excessive insulin release. The insulin causes fluctuations in blood sugar, which can lead to depression, anxiety, agitation, and fatigue. Simply eliminating this one food can profoundly impact your mental health in a positive way. Do not eat candy, cakes, cookies, pastry, ice cream, Twinkies, pies . . . You get the picture.

Grains can have a profound negative effect on brain functioning and are highly inflammatory. For all my patients with depression or any type of mental disorder, I recommend that they eat a grain-free diet—no wheat, rice, oats, bran, corn, barley, or spelt. There is abundant evidence that even whole grains can contribute to dementia, ADHD, depression, anxiety, chronic headaches, and more. For a complete and excellent review on this subject, I refer you to the book *Grain Brain* by Dr. David Perlmutter.

So we know what to avoid. But what then is left to eat? Plenty! Our brains thrive on healthy fats and cholesterol. Yes, cholesterol. Our brain is made up of 25% cholesterol.

We'll go into this more on the chapter on nutrition, but for now, know that the healthy oils include butter, coconut oil, palm oil, extra-virgin, dark olive oil, nut and seed oils, and avocado oil. Notice that I did not say canola, corn, soybean, vegetable, sunflower or safflower oil, or heaven forbid, margarine. These oils are highly inflammatory and can contribute to depression and heart disease.

Avoid highly processed foods and fast foods as much as possible. They are filled with chemicals, preservatives, MSG, high-fructose corn syrup, dyes, and a list of ingredients that are certainly not food. These also negatively impact our brain and can lead to a mind that is not clear and has difficulty making decisions. Also, avoid alcohol, as alcohol only worsens depression and kills brain cells.

Oftentimes, just cleaning up the diet is all that is necessary to treat the symptoms of depression. But other treatments include exercise—one of the strongest treatments for depression that exists. Maintaining good physical health can prevent depression from ever occurring in the first place. Regular exercise releases natural endorphins and increases the number of cells in the hippocampus—the area of the brain that is needed for short-term memory.

There are a number of nutrients that are critical for brain function and help alleviate depression. These include the following:

1. *Vitamin D or the sunshine vitamin.* The optimal level in the blood is between 70 and 90. Most of us have to take between 4,000 to 10,000 IU per day to meet this requirement. Vitamin D profoundly affects mood, and one study showed that those with low D levels were eleven times more likely to suffer from depression. Sunlight also helps depression significantly, perhaps in part to the vitamin D we get from the sun. Remember to always take D with food that contains fat or oil. I take mine with my fish oil in the morning.

2. *The B vitamins.* These are critical for energy and for brain functioning, especially vitamin B12. As we age, we tend to get deficient in B12, as our absorption of this vital nutrient decreases. When I have an older patient that complains of depression, I will always try vitamin B12 shots, once a week for eight weeks at first. In addition, I have them take B complex, one that is methylated. We'll learn more about it in the chapter on supplements. Basically, instead of folic acid, it should have methylfolate, and instead of cyanocobalamin, it should be methylcobalamin. These are highly absorbable and utilized more readily by the body.

3. *Omega-3 fats (such as fish oil).* These are critical. Optimal brain function critically relies on the omega-3s. The easiest way to get them is to take a pure-quality fish oil supplement at a dose of 2,000 mg twice a day. They are found in flax; in seafoods such as salmon, tuna, and halibut; and in nuts like walnuts. But it's hard to get sufficient amounts of omega-3s just from diet alone.

4. *Magnesium.* Most of us are deficient in this mineral, and being low in magnesium can cause depression, anxiety, insomnia, high blood pressure, and muscle cramps like charley horse. Most magnesium that is sold is magnesium oxide, which is poorly absorbed and causes diarrhea. Use magnesium

glycinate or chelate between 400 and 1,000 mg/day. I take mine right before bed to help with sleep.

5. *5-HTP.* This is the precursor for serotonin. In many studies, it works better than antidepressants.

6. *L-theanine.* It is an amino acid derivative. It helps the brain to release a neurotransmitter called GABA. It is very calming, it relieves anxiety, and it reduces stress. To be effective, L-theanine must be taken twice a day. Some patients have tried to take an actual GABA supplement, but it is hard to absorb and even harder to cross into the brain. You can get L-theanine in green tea.

7. *St. John's wort.* As an herbal remedy used for thousands of years, St. John's wort can alleviate mild to moderate depression. It must be a high-quality brand, or it will not be effective. The usual dose is 300 mg, three times daily.

8. *SAMe.* This has been shown to be very effective for some in treating depression. The typical dose is 800 mg twice a day. It is expensive but may be worth trying if other remedies have not helped. It works best with the B vitamins, and the combination of SAMe, B complex, and fish oil has turned many patients around.

9. *Essential oils.* These can also be useful for depression and are a simple thing to carry in the cab of your truck. The best ones for depression are bergamot, lavender, roman chamomile, orange, lemon, cinnamon, and ylang ylang.

Another tool for fighting depression is something called EFT or emotional freedom technique. EFT is a form of acupressure that's based on energy meridians that are used in acupuncture. Simple tapping with the fingertips is used to input kinetic energy onto specific locations on the body while you think about a specific problem and voice positive affirmations. The combination of tapping the energy meridians and voicing the positive affirmation works to clear emotional blocks, which is essential for optimal health and the healing of mental or physical disease. Go to YouTube and search for

EFT technique. It is quite simple and can be learned quickly. It can be effective for depression, anxiety, weight problems, healing from past trauma, and treatment of pain.

Another profound method for treating any mental disorder, and physical for that matter, is one called *The Emotion Code* by Dr. Bradley Nelson. It is a book I recommend more than any other for my patients that are interested in optimizing their health. You learn how to quickly release limiting emotions that are holding you back. Sometimes the emotions are inherited from our ancestors and, at other times, from our childhood. I have seen multiple instances where a blocked emotion being released caused a physical or mental pain to resolve completely.

Counseling or therapy can be profoundly helpful to those suffering from depression. Find someone that you can trust and are comfortable with and can help you gain insight into your background and situation. Finding the right therapist can be invaluable in your quest for emotional health.

Life is too short to not live fully and with the hope that even when things go wrong, there is light around the next corner. Don't let depression take that light from you. Men are that they might have joy. It is one of the reasons for our existence, and it is one that God wants each of us to experience.

Chapter 11

Fatigue

Tough times never last, but tough people do.

—Robert H. Schuller

Fatigue, or tiredness, is the number 1 complaint I always hear. At least half of every patient that walks in that door complains of being tired—tired when they wake up, tired in the afternoon, and certainly tired by the end of the day. The spring in their step has sprung, and it's often a struggle to simply get through the day.

Then at night, when sleep should give a welcome relief, it is often fragmented with frequent awakenings, a mind that won't turn off, or a body that is in pain and won't allow for a deep, restorative sleep. With fatigue comes a lower motivation, less willingness to take on extra projects or any projects at all for that matter, more brain fog, delayed reflexes, and less enthusiasm for life in general.

When you go to your doctor with a complaint of being tired all the time, the typical response will be to check some standard blood work, like a chemistry panel (CMP), a blood count for anemia (CBC), and one thyroid test called a TSH. Then if everything is normal, you'll be told that there's nothing wrong and you go exercise. You're just being lazy! Has this happened to you?

I'm here to tell you that if this is all that was done, only 5% of the workup was completed. There's another 95% that was overlooked as potential causes of fatigue, and we'll discuss these in more detail.

While fatigue is common the older we get, it should not be seen as inevitable and accepted that it's *normal* and, therefore, something we'll just have to live with. If you are tired all the time, it is a signal that the body is not working properly. It's a sign that the engine is malfunctioning and needs to be repaired. If every time you pushed on the accelerator of your truck you got a sluggish response, would you ignore it and say, "Oh, well, it's just getting older?" No, you would delve into the reason why and would take it to a mechanic or fix it yourself! In the same way, if your body is getting sluggish, we need to figure out why and fix the problem instead of just living with it.

There are many causes of fatigue, but we'll review the most common. These are the following:

Lack of sleep. The number 1 cause, by far, is insomnia. If you are not getting seven to eight hours of sleep per night, you are not being adequately rested. Common disruptions in sleep can be caused by OSA, as discussed earlier; too much caffeine; watching TV or using the computer before bedtime; an uncomfortable bed; and a mind that just won't turn off when you're trying to sleep. If you're an OTR driver, your sleeping cab should be your sanctuary. Do whatever it takes to make the bed and pillow comfortable. A memory foam topper works great and comes in many sizes. The MyPillow that is commonly advertised actually works wonders as well.

There are many medications for sleep. Most are addictive in nature and can cause grogginess in the morning, which is not a good thing if you're driving. Some may not be allowed for a driver having a CDL, such as benzodiazepines—Ativan (lorazepam), Valium (diazepam), Xanax (alprazolam), and Klonopin (clonazepam). Other addictive sedatives include Ambien (zolpidem) and Lunesta (eszopiclone). Both have the same warnings as the benzos: slower reaction times and daytime sedation. Nonaddictive meds for sleep include older drugs used for depression, including trazodone, doxepin, nortriptyline, and amitriptyline. Any and all prescription sedative drugs can be disqualifying on your DOT exam. Sometimes they will be approved with a note from the prescribing doctor stating that the driver is safe to operate a commercial vehicle while taking the medication.

There are long-term risks of sleep meds, including memory loss. All the sedative drugs are associated with slowing of brain waves in the frontal lobes, which contribute to the senior moments that are so common with aging. These can progress to dementia. Even over-the-counter antihistamines that are used for sleep, such as Benadryl, when taken nightly, has been linked to a higher risk of dementia.

Rather than risk your CDL license and risk your health, try natural approaches to insomnia. There are a variety of great natural supplements for insomnia. Most of us have heard of melatonin, but I find that often, melatonin by itself is not enough. It's commonly used in combination with other supplements, such as valerian root, magnesium, relora, GABA, L-theanine, and L-tryptophan.

Obesity. Any excess weight can contribute to fatigue. It takes a lot of work to carry around an extra twenty, fifty, or hundred pounds. Don't believe me? Just try picking up a fifty-pound bag and carrying it around all day. The cure, of course, is weight loss, and we'll talk about this in more detail in chapter.

Vitamin D deficiency. This is a common cause of tiredness. No matter if we live in the south or in northern climates, we are likely low in this critical vitamin. Take between 4,000 IU to 10,000 IU daily with food. I usually back off in the summertime, but any sunscreen you wear will block absorption of D. Supplementing with D can give you more energy, less joint pain, strengthen your immune system, and reduce risk of heart disease.

B vitamin deficiencies. The B vitamins are critical for energy production, and we absorb less B from our foods as we age. Also, if you're taking any antacids, they will block the absorption of the Bs, especially B12.

How do you know if you're low in B vitamins? Well, you can measure them in the blood, but a quicker, easier way is to look at your toes. If your second toe is longer than your big toe, you have a genetic defect in something called methylation or MTHFR. This means you do not process the B vitamins well and will tend to be lower in them, causing an increased risk of dementia, heart disease, cancer, anxiety, depression, and fatigue. It's quite common, seen in 40% of the population, and easily overcome by taking a methylated B vitamin.

Thyroid disease. The thyroid is the master regulator of our body and controls how much energy we make. This is such an important hormone that I will devote a whole chapter to it. Suffice it to say that hypothyroidism or low thyroid is often undiagnosed and leads to less energy, weight gain, chronic constipation, and dry skin. Most doctors don't know how to check for it adequately, and we'll discuss this in chapter.

Adrenal fatigue. This is very common in today's world. The adrenal glands sit on top of the kidneys and make cortisol, otherwise known as adrenaline. If the adrenals aren't producing cortisol properly, you'll suffer from low levels, leading to symptoms of low energy, difficulty getting up in the morning, and cravings of sugar and/or salt. The most common cause of low adrenals is intense emotional or physical stress, inflammation, low thyroid, and a poor diet. We'll devote an entire chapter on the adrenals, as you will never feel vibrant and well without healthy adrenals.

Depression. This typically causes a constant tiredness with low motivation. Please refer to the previous chapter.

Medications. Fatigue is a common side effect of multiple medications, so if you are taking anything that is either over-the-counter or prescribed, consider this as a cause.

Infections. As anyone who's had a cold can testify, getting an illness can sap all your energy, making it hard to even get out of bed. However, chronic fatigue can be caused by chronic infections such as mono, TB or tuberculosis, and a host of other viruses. Typically, there'll be other symptoms too, which make it easier to diagnose. Lyme disease is becoming more common and can be incredibly difficult to diagnose, as it hides out in our cells, evading detection. This disease can cause profound fatigue that goes on for years; if you are suspicious you have this illness, it is best to see a Lyme specialist.

Chronic illness. This category is vast and can include anything from cancer to heart disease, kidney disease, or lung disease. If the fatigue is lasting for longer than two months, make sure you get a complete physical to rule out any underlying problem.

Anemia. Low blood count means lower capacity to carry oxygen, which can cause a constant tiredness. The most common cause of anemia is heavy periods in women. If men have anemia, then colon cancer will need to be ruled out if their age is thirty or more. I'll never forget one male patient, aged thirty-five, who suffered from rectal bleeding off and on for two years. He was told that at his age, it was not cancer but likely a hemorrhoid. By the time I saw the patient and ordered his colonoscopy, he was diagnosed with metastatic colon cancer and died a few months later. Would he have survived if diagnosed two years earlier? Possibly, and that is tragic.

Diabetes. The more uncontrolled your diabetes, the higher your A1C and the more fatigued you will be. Why? Because the higher your A1C, the less oxygen-carrying capacity your blood cells have. You'll be more short of breath with exertion as well.

Toxins. We accumulate vast amount of toxins from the air we breathe to the foods we eat and even the products we apply on our skin and hair. I recommend a detoxification with the use of very specific supplements every six months to help clear out these toxins. On a daily basis, there are three simple things you can do: eat raw vegetables, drink six to eight cups of lemon water throughout the day every day, and wear a tourmaline gemstone bracelet or anklet. Tourmaline is a semiprecious mineral that generates an electric charge and emits negative ions and infrared energy. Electromagnetic radiation in the infrared range has many health effects, including detoxification, enhancing your immune system, improving circulation, and enhancing mood. It has so many positive benefits and is so easy to use. I wear my bracelet 24-7. It doesn't rust and does not decay. The price is normally $249 for one bracelet, but we are able to sell for $149 to allow more of you to benefit from this powerful mineral. See the supplement sections for more details.

If you are suffering from fatigue for more than two months, you've had your physical, and everything is *normal*, consider the following lab workup:

- Thyroid—TSH, free T3, free T4, and thyroid antibodies
- Vitamins B12, folate, D
- CMP—complete metabolic panel with liver and kidney function, electrolytes, protein, and calcium
- CBC—complete blood count for anemia
- UA—urine analysis to look for infection or protein in the urine, signifying kidney disease

Salivary cortisol levels. This is to rule out adrenal fatigue. The only accurate way to check the health of the adrenals is in the saliva, not blood. You have to spit in a tube four times in one day.

Sex hormones. Estrogens, progesterone, free and total testosterone— if these are abnormal, as in menopause for women or andropause for men, this can contribute to lower energy. We'll discuss this in much more detail in the next section.

A much more comprehensive assessment of nutritional status is done through a lab called Genova Diagnostics. Called a NutrEval, it measures all the vitamins, minerals, probiotics, omega-3/6/9, heavy metals, and digestive enzymes. Look at GDX.net.

Occasionally, I'll perform a urine heavy metal assessment and find that heavy metals are the cause of chronic fatigue.

Whatever the cause of your fatigue, even if it's been going on for years, you don't have to keep living with it. Find a doctor that knows functional medicine at WorldHealth.net. They'll give you the best chance at getting to the root of the problem and giving you your life back.

Chapter 12

JOINT AND BACK PAIN

Hustle until your haters ask if you're hiring.

Imagine living a life without pain. You can drive all day, lift heavy loads, throw them without difficulty, spring up from your chair without stiffness, walk briskly, and even run when you want. If this describes you, be grateful and go ahead and skip to the next section! But if not, keep reading.

Joint pain, low-back pain, and neck pain are common occurrences not only in your profession but also in many occupations. The typical response is to throw an over-the-counter medication at it, such as ibuprofen, Tylenol, or Aleve. These have minimal effect and can have multiple side effects.

Why do we develop back or joint pain? Degenerative arthritis begins to develop by age twenty, and by age forty, 90% of people will have signs of arthritis in their knees, even if they have no symptoms. The most common reason is obesity. It's a simple law of physics that the more weight you carry, the harder it is on your joints. Excess weight especially impacts the low back and knees.

But truck drivers in general have more back pain than most. To begin, sitting for prolonged periods can cause stiffness and back pain, and doing this for twenty years only compounds the problem.

Then there are back problems due to loading, unloading, and securing cargo. Oftentimes, these put tremendous pressure on the back, especially if proper lifting techniques aren't followed.

Two things can happen with the prolonged sitting and the physical activity involved with your job. First is spinal compression. The low back takes most of our weight, and the force is compounded in the lumbar spine or small of the back. This causes the discs between the vertebrae to flatten. The edges of the bone are no longer smooth, but they form spurs that can impinge on spinal nerves. As they are flattened, the discs can herniate, or protrude, putting pressure on the nerve. This can cause intense pain, sometimes radiating into the leg, and is known as sciatica.

Sciatica is caused by pressure on the sciatic nerve that runs from the low back to the buttocks and down the leg. The pain is often felt deep in the buttocks and radiates into the back of the leg, extending past the knee in most cases, even to the foot, depending on which nerve is affected.

Strains and muscle spasms of the back are very common and can be treated with ice, heat, massage, and occasional chiropractic care.

But how do you prevent the back pain from occurring in the first place? Supporting the low back is key, and the simplest way to protect the back is by using a pillow in the small of your back while you drive. You'll be surprised at how effective this can be. Also, make sure that your truck seats have well-supported springs to absorb vibration and decrease the force delivered to the back.

Another simple maneuver you can do to reduce back pain is to decompress the spine. You can do this by simply squatting. This will cause the space between the vertebrae to open and decompress. With your heels together, knees apart, and feet flat, squat as low as you can go. Try to remain there for twenty to thirty seconds at a time. You can hold on to something in front of you if need to keep from falling over. Ideally, squatting should be done every two hours, but knowing the reality of the long-haul truck driver, do this at least three times a day. You can do it in the cab of your truck without anyone seeing. (See pic.)

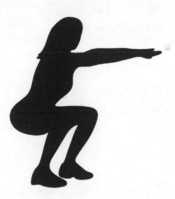

Besides back pain, there's all the other joints that start to hurt, especially the knees. Knee pain is so common with truck drivers that it is seen as an occupational hazard. It comes from getting in and out of the truck, walking, and lifting heavy loads. I've been told by drivers that the left knee is usually the worst because of the clutch. And as discussed before, the more excessive weight you carry, the more wear and tear on the knees.

A common condition that affects truck drivers is patellar tendonitis, otherwise known as jumper's knee. The patellar tendon is a thick tendon that connects the kneecap to the tibia or shinbone. It acts to straighten the knee and is necessary for kicking. The tendon can become painful with overuse, repeated stress, and strain on the tendon, causing it to become inflamed. The first symptom is usually pain underneath the kneecap. It occurs with activity, especially climbing or going down stairs. Treatment involves icing the patellar tendon for twenty minutes a night and using an anti-inflammatory cream directly over the tendon. Aspercreme is available over the counter. Use it twice a day. You can also get your doctor to prescribe ketoprofen 10% cream from a compounding pharmacy. It works great. You apply it twice a day, and it's absorbed through the skin, having a direct anti-inflammatory effect over the tendon.

Natural anti-inflammatories are very important to reduce the pain, inflammation and to help build up the cartilage that is being lost with aging. The best ones have the following:

Glucosamine sulfate. This is one of the most popular supplements for joint health and helps your body rebuild and maintain joint tissues such as cartilage, tendons, and ligaments. It is a natural anti-inflammatory. It also is used for autoimmune disease and helps heal the gut lining and rebuild tissue and stronger bones following fractures or injuries. Dosage is 500 mg to 1,500 mg twice a day, and it works best with other joint supplements. Glucosamine must be the *sulfate* form to be effective to rebuild cartilage.

MSM (methylsulfonylmethane). What the heck is that? It's a simply wonderful supplement that contains sulfur and is used to lower inflammation, improve the immune function, and help with detoxification. It is especially popular as a supplement to treat arthritis, or degenerative joint disease, since it helps form connective tissue and repair joints, tendons, and ligaments. Many studies have shown that it decreases joint inflammation, helps to rebuild collagen, and improves flexibility. Joint pain, stiffness, and knee and back pain can be helped with MSM. As an added benefit, it also improves collagen production in the skin to help make our skin look more youthful. Dosage is 500 mg once to twice a day.

Boswelia. This is a natural anti-inflammatory. It has been shown to reduce joint pain by 32% to 65%. Dosage is 100 mg/day.

Turmeric and ginger. Both reduce pain, inflammation, and stiffness in both rheumatoid arthritis and degenerative arthritis (osteoarthritis). It may also help to prevent breast, colon, and prostate cancer. Use turmeric and ginger in your cooking as much as possible. Dosage is 75 mg/day.

Rosemary. It has been used for thousands of years for its strong anti-inflammatory properties. Taken orally, the usual dose is 75 mg/day. Rosemary is very easy to grow, and you can brew a homemade tea with rosemary, ginger, mint, and lemon, sweetened with stevia if desired. Let it steep for half an hour. Rosemary essential oil is great to carry with you in the truck. You can use it on a sore joint, rub it on your temples if you have a headache, massage a few drops on your chest and throat for a cough, dilute in water and use as a mouthwash, and inhale directly from the bottle to increase mental acuity.

Niacinamide (vitamin B3). It is not considered an anti-inflammatory. It triggers actual repair of the joint surfaces that leads to dramatic reduction in joint pain and inflammation. Niacinamide also has antiaging properties by helping to silence the aging gene. It improves glucose metabolism and stimulates cellular energy metabolism. The optimal dose is 250 mg to 500 mg every three hours. It has a short half-life and has to be taken frequently. At a dose of 3,000 mg daily, you'll get the joint relief and the antiaging effect.

Quercetin. This is a powerful antioxidant found in colorful foods, such as leafy greens, tomatoes, berries, and purple and red vegetables. It helps fight free radicals and has strong anti-inflammatory effects. There may also be cancer-fighting abilities with quercetin. You can get plenty of this antioxidant with eating colorful vegetables daily (french fries are not colorful!), and you can take it in a capsule form, from 50 mg to 500 mg/day.

Cetyl myristoleate (CMO). This is an oil found in fish and dairy butter. It acts as an anti-inflammatory and helps lubricate the joint. Dosage is 40 mg/day.

Omega-3s. I can't say enough about the omega-3s, most commonly found in fish oil. They are widely used to reduce inflammation, and in joint pain, they may help to keep the joints lubricated. They work especially well with glucosamine. Dose is 3,000 mg/day.

Bromelain. This is an enzyme found in pineapples and acts as a natural anti-inflammatory. It's often used in combination with other ingredients found above, but you can also get it by eating fresh pineapple.

Emotional component. Addressing the emotional component of arthritis is often overlooked but extremely important. I won't delve into this in detail, but suffice it to say that degenerative joint pain is often associated with blocked emotions of irritation and frustration. The severity of the problem depends on how intense these emotions are, what the underlying emotional trauma was that caused it in the first place, and at what age. These emotions can get blocked and stuck in our joints, leading to inflammation and the degenerative changes seen. Read *The Emotion Code* by Dr. Nelson for more information, and this will empower you to release these emotions on your own and to help transform this energy for good.

Stem cell therapy. The newest and most profound treatment for arthritis is stem cell therapy. I'll discuss this more in chapter, but the bottom line is that stem cells have the potential to reverse the arthritis in your joint and regrow cartilage. We use stem cells harvested from umbilical cord blood after birth and inject it in the affected joint. Stem cells have the power to become any cell, and when injected in a joint with arthritis, it will develop into cartilage cells, suppress inflammation, and release proteins that slow down cartilage degeneration. This procedure is done in the office and is not covered by insurance. That being said, I have seen patients on the verge of a knee replacement able to cancel surgery and walk again with minimal pain. Even though the injection is not covered by insurance, they actually saved money by not having to take time off work to have surgery or pay their deductible.

Gluten-free diet. I can't tell you how many times I've seen patients' joint pain improve as soon as they eliminated gluten from their diet. For some, complete elimination of all grains was required. They'll say that as soon as they started eating gluten, the joint pain returned. Gluten can be highly inflammatory, and removing it from the diet can improve joint pain, memory, irritable bowel syndrome, and fatigue. It has a terrible side effect: weight loss.

As you can see, there are many ways to treat arthritis, but the most important thing is to get to the root cause. Clean up the diet, try eliminating gluten to see if this is a factor, eat plenty of colorful vegetables, remove any underlying emotional blocks, and take a natural anti-inflammatory. This combination will give you powerful results and, at the same time, reduce your risk for heart disease, diabetes, stroke, and cancer.

Section Two

HEALTHY HORMONES

Vision without action is daydream. Action without vision is nightmare.

Chapter 13

TESTOSTERONE

We age because our hormones decline; our hormones don't decline because we age.

Mike was fifty-two years old, and over the last few years, he noticed changes to his body he attributed to middle age—weight gain around the middle, no longer just love handles anymore; snoring; more tiredness and lower motivation; less enthusiasm for life, often choosing to come home after work and sit in his recliner in front of the TV where he fell asleep; erectile dysfunction, being unable to sustain an erection and lower libido overall; higher cholesterol; and now his blood pressure was creeping up. Now his wife was complaining that he was getting grumpy.

His wife finally made him see his doctor, who diagnosed him with depression, high cholesterol, obesity, and prediabetes. He was told to start a med for depression, one for cholesterol, metformin for the prediabetes, and oh yeah, lose weight. He was just told to eat less and start exercising for one hour a day.

He left there feeling even more irritable and depressed than when he went in. Feeling he should start the meds as directed by his doctor, he took them for four weeks and felt worse than ever. Now his muscles hurt all over, his fatigue was ten times worse, the metformin caused gas and diarrhea, and the antidepressant had no effect on his mood but instead made his ED and lack of libido more pronounced than before. He tried to exercise, but the muscle pain made it nearly impossible, not to mention the profound fatigue.

When he complained to his family doctor on the follow-up appointment, he was told to continue the course, and things would improve with time. As far as the antidepressant, instead of stopping it, the medication was doubled.

But instead of following doctor's orders, he decided to take matters into his own hands. *There must be a better way!* He started researching his symptoms online and found multiple articles on the effects of testosterone and, particularly, what happens as it begins to decline.

Deciding to seek a second opinion, Mike saw me in the office. After a complete workup, I diagnosed him with low testosterone, or low T, an underactive thyroid, adrenal fatigue, and high estrogen. He was also vitamin D deficient. I noticed his second toe was longer than his big toe and knew he had a defect in methylation, which caused his B vitamins to be lower.

The treatment was to fix the underlying biochemical defects and to taper him off all his meds that were causing nothing but side effects. I started him on 10,000 IU of vitamin D daily, 3,000 mg/day of fish oil, a methylated B complex twice a day, methylated B12 shots for a total of six given once a week, and 100 mg of CoQ10 a day because of his deficiency caused by his cholesterol med. Then testosterone replacement using bioidentical testosterone at a dose of 50 mg/day was given as a transdermal cream that is rubbed on in the morning.

Next he was prescribed an antiestrogen drug called anastrazole to take three days a week. It was no use prescribing testosterone if he was going to keep shunting it over to estrogen! Twenty-five milligrams a day of DHEA was supplemented as an antiaging hormone to help even further with libido and to slow the aging process. A bioidentical type of thyroid called Nature-Throid was prescribed, and he also started on adrenal supplements to take in the morning and at noon.

The follow-up three months later was remarkable. He had lost twenty pounds, was actually exercising again, and was noticing an increase in muscle mass. His energy was back, and with it came a sharp mind and motivation and enthusiasm for his work. His love life improved greatly, and the depression, irritability, and grumpiness had been completely resolved. He no longer snored, much to the wife's delight. Blood work showed his cholesterol had improved, thyroid function was back to normal, and the prediabetes had resolved, with his A1C dropping from 5.9 to 5.5.

Is this a unique case? Not at all. By far, in men, the most common cause of depression, fatigue, weight gain, lower libido, snoring, high cholesterol, and ED is a low testosterone. Remember the movie *Grumpy Old Men*? That's what happens to men as they age and lose their testosterone. They become grumpy, fat, irritable, lazy, and lose that spark of life. And as the estrogen increases, they develop the all-too-common man boobs. See men with that? Then you know that their estrogen is too high. I've seen men with their estrogen higher than their testosterone!

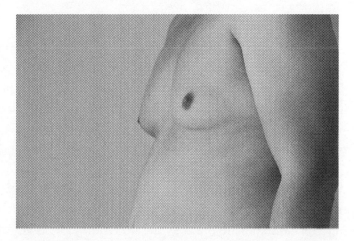

Testosterone is made in the testicles at the time of puberty, and it contributes to muscle mass, hair growth, a deeper voice, increased bone density, and emotional health and drive. Testosterone begins to decline at age thirty, but I've seen it low in as young as eighteen years of age. There are many reasons for this, including the increased use of chemicals that interfere with testosterone production.

Many of these chemicals are endocrine disruptors and lower testosterone while increasing estrogen in men. These chemicals are everywhere, including household cleaners, the BPA in plastics, personal hygiene products, Roundup, pesticides, toothpaste, the lining of aluminum cans, and dairy products, just to name a few. Why dairy? Growth-promoting hormones and estrogen-mimicking chemicals are added to commercial dairy products.

Symptoms of low testosterone include

- fatigue, less motivation, less drive;
- erectile dysfunction, lower sex drive, less ejaculation;
- less muscle mass, more fat accumulation, especially abdominal;
- joint pain and stiffness, muscles being sore more easily with exercise, decreased response to exercise;
- depression, irritability, and insomnia; and
- brain fog or *fuzzy* brain.

The male brain is highly dependent on testosterone, and as the level begins to decline, they commonly complain of brain fog. The brain processing speed just isn't as fast as it used to be, short-term memory is affected, and there is less drive and motivation. The declining levels seen with age is sometimes termed as andropause, as opposed to the woman's menopause. The effects can be just as dramatic.

Testosterone affects every organ system in the body. Its effects are widespread. It helps maintain muscle mass and strength. It also is responsible for bone density, and as the levels decline, this puts men at risk of osteoporosis and muscle atrophy. It stimulates red blood cell formation and reduces risk of anemia.

Testosterone replacement is safe and can provide dramatic benefits while slowing the aging process. Benefits are seen throughout the entire male body, including the following:

- Lowers risk of heart disease by 30% to 50%. Testosterone lowers inflammation, which then lowers risk of heart attacks, strokes, angina, and sudden death. One of the mechanisms could be an increase in nitric oxide production, which improves cardiovascular health. If this was all testosterone did, it would be reason enough to prescribe, and if there were any drug that was able to do this, it would sell billions.
- Lowers risk of dementia and possibly other brain-related disorders such as Parkinson's disease by 20%. Remember, the male brain depends on testosterone, which has been shown to improve cerebral blood flow.
- Improves bone density and helps prevent osteoporosis.
- Improves muscle strength even without exercise, but when exercise is added, there is marked improvement by increasing protein synthesis.
- Improves sexual performance and libido.
- Reduces abdominal visceral fat.
- Slows down the rate of aging.
- Fights depression and helps prevent its occurrence in the first place. In any middle-aged male, before starting an antidepressant, always measure testosterone levels and replace if needed.
- Controls the distribution of facial fat. A man with a chiseled and more angular face has high testosterone levels.
- Increases metabolism. High testosterone levels directly inhibit the formation of new fat cells and increases the metabolic rate, allowing you to eat more and not gain weight.

Studies have also shown that men that are hospitalized for any reason, those on testosterone, have a decreased risk of death, are readmitted less often, and are able to be discharged from the hospital earlier.

But what about the prostate? There is a misconception that testosterone therapy can cause prostate cancer, or if you have a small tumor, it can cause it to grow quickly or that the hormone can increase a condition called BPH (benign prostatic hypertrophy). Basically, BPH means an enlarged prostate.

BPH occurs commonly as men age, where the prostate can enlarge and put pressure on the urethra—the tube from the bladder to the tip of the penis. This makes it difficult to urinate and can decrease the force of the urinary stream. Oftentimes, men will complain of urinating smaller amounts and getting up in the night to urinate.

Does testosterone treatment cause an enlarged prostate, or if you already have BPH, can it make it worse? Let me put the issue to rest. Absolutely not! Testosterone does *not* cause an enlarged prostate. If it did, men in their twenties with raging testosterone levels would all have BPH. When does the prostate start to enlarge? After age fifty, when men are experiencing significant decline in their testosterone levels. If anything, taking testosterone will often help shrink an enlarged prostate.

How about prostate cancer? I want to be very clear on this. Testosterone does *not* cause prostate cancer. Again, if it did, men in their teens and twenties would all have prostate cancer. But instead, the cancer starts to occur after age fifty, when levels of testosterone are declining. The myth that testosterone causes prostate cancer was based on only *one* patient in 1941 who was given testosterone and reported that it caused his prostate cancer to grow. They measured a blood level of acid phosphatase to make this determination. Multiple other patients found that testosterone administration caused no prostate cancer progression. Some men experienced improvement, with less bone pain.

Since then, many studies have shown no correlation with prostate cancer. Indeed, some studies giving testosterone to men with prostate cancer have been shown to reduce the aggressiveness of the tumor.

And while we're on this subject, let's talk about the PSA blood test, which is used as a screen for prostate cancer. While there is currently a lot of controversy regarding PSA, most doctors will still start to screen for it at age fifty. Here's the most important thing to remember. If you keep your PSA less than 1.5, your risk of prostate cancer is extremely low. If your PSA is between 1.5 and 4, your risk is fifteen times higher than those with PSA less than 1.5.

If you have a PSA more than 1.5, the best test at this point is something called 4Kscore (4KScore.com). Covered by insurance and Medicare, it's a simple blood test that will help differentiate if there is prostate cancer, and if there is, it is likely to be indolent or aggressive. If there's a low risk, you can usually just follow your levels with time, rather than agree to the invasive procedure of a prostate biopsy.

When prescribing testosterone, there are three options. One is a cream that is absorbed through the skin, another is pellets that are injected under the skin and last for four to five months, and another is injections. Testosterone should always be bioidentical, not synthetic. *Bioidentical* means the chemical structure is the same as what your body produces. Drug companies cannot patent bioidentical forms, so they have to change something about it so that it does not have the same effects. Synthetic testosterone includes brands such as AndroGel or Testim, which cost anywhere from $200 to $450 a month, or Depo-Testosterone injections. Depo-Testosterone has been implicated in liver cancer and increases inflammation, not decreases.

Bioidentical testosterone is made by a compounding pharmacy and is identical in structure to what your body naturally makes. It's far safer and far cheaper, averaging around $40 to $50 a month.

When I'm measuring a man's testosterone, I always measure it at 8:00 AM—the time of peak production. Estrogens must also be ordered, as estrone and estradiol. This is because as men age, they often convert some testosterone to estrogen. And the more belly fat you have, the more this process occurs.

Once I have the lab, I'll prescribe based on the results. Usually, we'll try testosterone in a cream first as it's easiest. The dose can range anywhere from 25 mg to 100 mg and is given once a day. It's applied first thing in the morning on an area of the body that doesn't have a lot of hair, like the inner arms, inner thighs, or shoulders. Don't apply it on the abdomen or genital area.

If the estrogen is high, we'll need to lower that, as it does no good to give testosterone to just convert it to estrogen. An easy way to bring it down is with a medication that is an antiestrogen called anastrozole or armidex. The dose is 1 mg. Take half a tab one to three times per week. Other ways to lower estrogen is with 50 mg zinc, 320 mg/day of saw palmetto, and something called chrysin, which is added to the testosterone cream. Your doctor will need to monitor your estradiol level; it should not get too low. Optimal estradiol is 25–50 pg/ml. Some estrogen is needed by men as it's necessary for brain, heart, bone, and sexual function.

If estrogen is too high, this can increase risk of prostate cancer, cause insulin resistance predisposing to diabetes, and cause the all-too-familiar man boobs. The fat buildup in the breasts is very resistant to treatment, including weight loss. We've used a procedure called CoolSculpting to freeze and kill the fat cells there. I'll discuss this more in the weight loss chapter.

There's another form of testosterone called DHT. It is a stronger form of testosterone and is needed for erectile function and muscle building. It can cause hair loss and is associated with BPH, but it is not prostate cancer.

Testosterone cream works great for most men and is absorbed well. You'll form a little more DHT with the cream, so if BPH symptoms start, take the saw palmetto or other prostate formula. The main negative with the cream is the risk of cross contamination—exposing your wife, kids, or grandkids to the cream. Once you apply it, if someone touches that area for up to four hours later, you can transfer some of the cream to them. Don't touch the cream with your hands either, or then the faucet and sink will be contaminated. Cover the area of skin with your clothes, and you should be fine.

To measure levels of testosterone when using transdermal cream, you'll need to do a saliva test. This is a test where you simply spit in a tube that is sent to a lab, and it can give measurements of testosterone, estrogen, progesterone, and DHEA. The mistake many doctors who have not been trained in this field make is measuring blood levels of testosterone when using the cream and writing their prescription based on these levels. I once had a man come into my office using 800 mg of testosterone a day! Why? His doctor was drawing his blood, which kept coming back low, so continued to increase his dose. Eight hundred milligrams is extremely high, and too much of a good thing can be deadly. We had to slowly taper it over several months, and he began to feel less aggressive.

Testosterone can decrease the size of the testicles by up to 25%, as the testicles reduce the production of the hormone and, therefore, size decreases. It can also cause infertility with a decrease in sperm production. You would think it would be opposite, but it isn't. So in a young male who wants to maintain fertility, giving testosterone is not a good option.

In this case, we would use either Clomid and or hCG. Both of these work well in younger men who want to maintain fertility and get the body to increase its production of the hormone. The usual dose for hCG is 1,000 to 2,000 IU twice a week. You can use hCG in conjunction with testosterone to decrease the risk of reducing testicular size. Before trying hCG, you need to measure two hormones called FSH and LH. If these are high, it is unlikely hCG will be effective.

The next option for testosterone is pellets. These are small pellets that are inserted under the skin in the buttock area that slowly release testosterone over four to five months. They have to be replaced every three to five months. You can feel when they're wearing off. They are generally a more expensive option, but the benefit is, there's no risk of contamination of the hormone. And once they're in, you don't have to worry about it for several months.

A very common route of administration of testosterone is injection. The old way of giving the shots was once every two weeks. This is no longer recommended, as it caused blood levels to be too high for several days after the shot and too low before the next shot was due. Therefore, the patient complained of being too aggressive or anxious after the shot and in a slump before the next shot.

Now we recommend twice-a-week shots, giving a lower dosage with each injection. This causes much less variability in blood levels, and most men respond to it very well. The usual dose is giving testosterone cypionate at 25 mg to 75 mg twice a week. Notice that I said testosterone cypionate, *not* Depo-Testosterone. The shot is usually given in the lateral thigh, and you'll need to be shown how to give the injections yourself. You can do this on the road. Just be sure to carry enough supplies—syringes, needles, and a sharp box to put the needles in once used.

The advantage of injections versus cream is that levels can be easily measured in the blood. When measuring the testosterone level, always draw the lab the day *before* your next shot is due.

Testosterone can have profound effects on our health, your well-being, your attitude, and your love life. It has minimal risks, and every aging male may benefit from this hormone. If you have any of the symptoms above, don't walk; run to the nearest doctor and have your levels measured.

In summary, for the lab, free and total testosterone, estrone, estradiol, DHEA-S lab should be drawn at 8:00 AM. The optimal levels for total testosterone are 500–750; free testosterone, 15–25; estradiol, 25–50; DHEA, 200 or higher. For medication, use 25–100 mg/day of testosterone cream or 25–75 mg of testosterone cypionate twice weekly or 1,000–2,000 IU of hCG twice a week or 75–100 mg of pellets every three to four months. For antiestrogen, use half a tab of 1 mg anastrozole one to three times per week.

Chapter 14

PMS AND MENOPAUSE

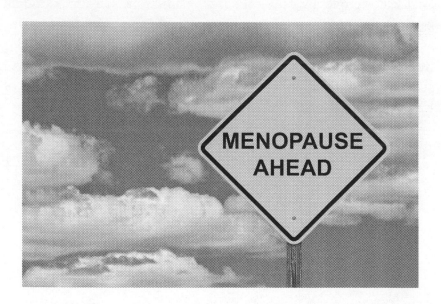

Everything you do now is for your future. Think about that.

The last chapter was for the men. This chapter is for the ladies. I'll admit, I never had a lot of interest in this topic until I approached that phase of life. Then, all of a sudden, it mattered to me a great deal! But the training I had in medical school failed to teach me about this topic or how to appropriately treat it or if you should even treat at all. I had to go back to school, and I eventually obtained a second board certification in antiaging and regenerative medicine. That is where I learned the ins and outs of prescribing hormone therapy and using bioidentical hormones for both women and men.

The average age of menopause is fifty-two, but the process starts at least ten years earlier. Past age thirty-five, the female hormone progesterone begins to decline. This often leads to the symptoms of PMS or premenstrual syndrome.

Have you ever known someone with PMS? Anywhere from a day to a week before the menstrual cycle, the symptoms can start—irritability, bloating, fluid retention, headaches, emotional lability, anxiety, insomnia, and increased carbohydrate cravings. Oftentimes, the periods will start to get heavier and last longer, with painful cramping.

Go to a traditional doctor with these complaints, and you'll be given an antidepressant and possibly birth control pills. Maybe you'll be given a water pill to take for the swelling and a sleeping pill to use as needed.

None of these are the solution, and all have the potential to make things worse. The underlying problem is progesterone—the lack of it.

Progesterone is a woman's friend. It is calming, relieves anxiety, helps us sleep soundly, lowers joint pain, helps with bone density, and lowers the risk of breast cancer. If you have a lot more estrogen than progesterone, you are estrogen dominant, which will increase your risk of breast cancer. Try a little bioidentical progesterone cream, which you can get at any health food store or on Amazon. Use 20 mg on the last two weeks of your cycle.

The first day of your menstrual cycle is day 1. So assuming your period is every twenty-eight days, start the progesterone cream on days 14–28. I have some women that only need it the last week, on days 21–28, and others that feel so much better with it that they'll use more.

On days 1–5, use none.

On days 6–11, use once a day.

On days 12–28, apply twice a day.

You'll know if you're using too much if your breasts start to get tender. Then back off to half the amount.

Hot flashes can start in your forties from the lack of progesterone. Often the treatment is simply the progesterone cream, and it is a safe and easy thing to try.

But once menopause occurs, then it won't be enough. Menopause is defined as a lack of a period for one year and as the ovaries no longer releasing any eggs. The production of estrogen from the ovaries dramatically drops, which can lead to more hot flashes.

If any of you have ever experienced a hot flash, you'll never forget. It's a feeling of intense heat, or a flushing, that can occur only in the face or the entire upper body. Red blotches can occur, and you'll want to fan yourself or, perhaps, throw yourself into a snow bank! Night sweats can also occur, interrupting your sleep and causing you to sleep with a fan every night.

Not every woman has hot flashes; 20% never experience a single one. They are the lucky ones.

Some studies have shown that women with severe hot flashes have a higher risk of earlier heart disease. Why? Because the hot flashes imply that there is inflammation raging throughout your arteries. And believe me, if you've ever had a hot flash, it feels like there's fire burning inside and coursing through every artery.

After menopause, both estrogen and progesterone are low, and testosterone may be either up or down. In some women, the testosterone is normal or high for the first few years after menopause. For others, it's low or has been low for years.

Pamela has been driving for twenty-four years, from Spokane to Seattle and back four days a week. The job suits her, as it allows her to be home in the evening and on weekends for her family. She's always enjoyed a good relationship with her husband, but now things seem to have changed. Since going through menopause two years ago, she is still having hot flashes and night sweats, and the insomnia is dragging her down. Because of the lack of sleep, she's more irritable and finds herself getting short with the kids. She's also noticed her metabolism has changed, and twenty pounds seem to have come on overnight.

Other changes have been happening in the bedroom. Her complete lack of sex drive has put a damper on her sex life, and when she is intimate with her husband, the vaginal dryness is painful. Lubrication like K-Y isn't enough anymore.

Finally getting fed up enough to do something about it, Pamela decides to go to her doctor. Dr. Mainstream tells her the bad news. She's menopausal and will have to learn to deal with it. An antidepressant is offered (that seems to be the answer to everything), and when Pamela asks about hormones, she is flatly told no. They cause cancer, heart attacks, and are downright evil! But if they cause all these things and are so bad for you, then why don't twenty-year-olds all have cancer and heart attacks? Dr. Mainstream stutters a bit, gives her the script for Prozac, and says to pay on the way out.

If this is your experience, I have some exciting news. This does not have to be you anymore!

When I saw Pamela, who came to me after the advice from a friend, I measured all her hormones, including thyroid. She was thirty pounds overweight, her blood pressure was borderline, and she had prediabetes. Her estrogens, progesterone, and testosterone were all low. So was the powerful powerhouse and antiaging hormone, DHEA. Thyroid was borderline. It was not low enough to start treatment but on the way. I started bioidentical hormones, DHEA, and a thyroid supplement to wake the thyroid up. She was also prescribed estrogen in a vaginal cube to insert three nights per week. Other supplements such as B vitamins, a whole food multivitamin, fish oil, and vitamin D were also started.

Three months later in follow-up, she was a new woman. Her hot flashes had been completely resolved, and she was sleeping again. Her relationship with her husband improved. The libido wasn't completely back to what she considered as normal, but it was enough to make the relationship happy and healthy again. Vaginal dryness was gone, and she now reduced the estriol vaginal cube to one to two times per week. Her weight was down thirteen pounds, and she found she wasn't craving the carbs like before.

Is this a unique case? No, it is not! The metabolic changes that occur at the time of menopause are profound. The rate of aging accelerates without our hormones, and the weight piles on easily. The average weight gain when a woman goes through menopause is twenty pounds, but I often see much more. And though the weight goes on quickly, it comes off slowly, as many women can attest.

At the same time, blood pressure is creeping up and insulin levels are rising, which, of course, contributes to more weight gain. Arteries are getting stiffer, leading to a condition called endothelial dysfunction, which leads to earlier heart disease. The ligaments, tendons, and cartilages around joints are losing their elasticity; and arthritis is accelerating.

Hormone imbalances are at the roots of many problems and cause chronic disease. But the good news is that the imbalances can be corrected with bioidentical hormone replacement therapy or BHRT.

Women are more complicated than males, and instead of just testosterone to measure and correct, we need to balance estrogens and progesterone.

Estrogens are the main female hormone, and there are three types.

1. *E1 (estrone).* This estrogen is the main one we make after menopause, and it's primarily made in our fat cells. It has been implicated in breast cancer, and when prescribing BHRT, we therefore never use E1 in the prescription.
2. *E2 (estradiol).* This is the strongest estrogen and is responsible for protecting the bones from osteoporosis, or thinning, and protects us from heart disease. Estradiol is the main estrogen that relieves us from hot flashes. It is also critical for brain functioning, and after menopause and its decline, women complain of brain fog and mental fuzziness. We use this in concentrations of 20% to 50% estradiol.
3. *E3 (estriol).* This is the weakest estrogen. It is much higher in pregnancy than in nonpregnant women. It has powerful anti-inflammatory effects and gut-healing properties. It has been shown in some studies to help protect against breast cancer. We use this in concentrations of 50% to 80%.

The next important female hormone is progesterone. This hormone is vitally important and may help prevent breast cancer. The main mistake I see traditional doctors make is the statement "If you've had a hysterectomy, you don't need progesterone." And the second biggest lie is that Provera, or the generic medroxyprogesterone, is the same as progesterone.

Both of these statements are not only utterly false but also harmful! To say that if you don't have a uterus, you don't need progesterone is ridiculous. Progesterone receptors are found throughout the body, and it is critical for so many things, including the following:

- Regulates blood sugar and helps prevent diabetes
- Calms and relieves anxiety, allowing for a deeper sleep
- Needed for bone protection and stimulates new bone growth
- Acts as a natural diuretic and reduces water retention
- Inhibits breast tissue overgrowth and helps protect the breasts from cancer
- Prevents excessive buildup of the uterine lining
- Enhances the effect of thyroid hormones
- Increases metabolism and promotes fat loss

So as you can see, it doesn't matter if you have a uterus or if you do not. You need progesterone to balance the estrogen and for the many health benefits it provides.

Now, as for the false statement that Provera is the same as progesterone, nothing could be farther from the truth. Provera is not bioidentical and is highly inflammatory. It causes great many side effects, such as bloating, headache, weight gain, joint pain, and higher risk of heart disease. Do not allow your doctor to ever prescribe this drug. If he must prescribe a progesterone that is made from the drug companies, he can prescribe Prometrium. It comes in 100 mg or 200 mg tabs and is taken at night.

Testosterone is extremely important for women as well as men. The levels must be measured, though, to know whether to prescribe or not. If the levels are low, most women will need between 0.5 mg and 4 mg a day. You'll know you're getting too much if you start getting acne and facial hair growth.

BHRT in women can be given in four ways.

Transdermal cream. This is applied twice a day. BHRT in a cream has a half-life of twelve hours; hence, it is applied twice a day. Most women apply the cream on the upper inner arms or on the thighs. Rotate the sites. Don't use it on the same spot every day. And know that if someone touches the area where it's applied, they can be exposed to some of the cream. That's not a good thing for men or children.

The main mistake doctors make on prescribing BHRT in a cream is that they check the levels in the blood. The blood will always read too low when using a cream and cannot be used. The only accurate way to check levels in this case is in the saliva. We send the kits home with the patient, and they are not covered by insurance in most cases.

Pellets. These are implanted just under the skin in the buttock area. They last between three to five months and have to be replaced as they wear off. It's a more expensive option and more invasive.

BLA tabs. These are a method most are not aware of. BLA stands for bio-lymphatic absorption. This is the only safe way to take estrogen by mouth, as it bypasses the liver's first-pass metabolism. It's not metabolized through the liver, but it is slowly absorbed into the lymphatic system over eight hours. This method is easy, convenient, and about the same cost as the cream. Levels can be measured in the blood, and the lab should be drawn five to eight hours after the pill is taken.

Sublingual troche. This is less commonly used. This is a soft tablet that dissolves under the tongue. It doesn't always give steady serum levels, and the taste can be unpleasant. The cost is about the same as the cream, and levels can be measured in the blood.

A common question from women is, How long can I safely stay on the hormones? The answer, quite simply, is indefinitely. There is no reason to stop them as we age because as soon as they're discontinued, all the benefits are reversed. Aging accelerates; risk of heart disease, dementia, and bone loss increases; and hot flashes may occur again. Why stop them at all? Let's fool the body into thinking it's younger than it really is. And as an aside, they do not affect the DOT in any way.

So if you want to feel younger, more energetic, sexier, healthier, and maintain your weight more easily, then bioidentical hormones are for you.

Chapter 15

THYROID

A diamond is a chunk of coal that did well under pressure.

The thyroid is a butterfly-shaped gland that sits just below the Adam's apple in the neck. (See pic.) It's an innocuous little gland and looks innocent enough. You'd never know what power this gland has.

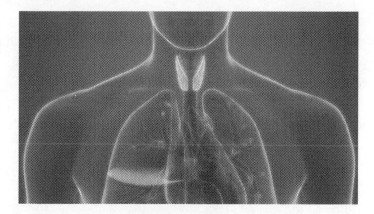

The thyroid is the master regulator of the entire body. It controls the metabolic rate in every cell of the body and how many calories you burn each day. Symptoms of low thyroid include

- hair loss and the lateral third of the eyebrows thinning;
- fatigue;

- weight gain;
- constipation;
- dry skin and brittle nails;
- cold hands and feet;
- high cholesterol (the metabolism of cholesterol is controlled by the thyroid);
- slow speech, slow movements, slow thoughts; and
- low blood pressure.

Most doctors do not know how to properly diagnose a low thyroid, known as hypothyroidism. If you go to your doctor with a complaint of tiredness, most often they'll check one thyroid lab called the TSH. And they'll miss 50% or more of thyroid disease.

To properly diagnose hypothyroidism, the following should be ordered: TSH, free T3, free T4, and thyroid antibodies.

T3 is the active form of thyroid, and it controls our metabolism and how much energy each cell produces. The free T3 is the unbound, active form of T3 and is much more important than total T3. Optimal levels of FT3 are between 3.5 and 4.5. Most labs show that *normal* FT3 is 2.0–4.5, but if your FT3 were in the 2s, you would most likely complain of fatigue and difficulty losing weight.

One of the most common causes of a low T4 to T3 conversion is stress and the stress hormone—cortisol. High cortisol suppresses this conversion and can lead to hypothyroidism. Another cause in women is a high estrogen when taking estrogen orally or with birth control pills. Estrogen can cause more of the T3 to be bound, making it unavailable to use. The only treatment for this is to detoxify and clear out the estrogen.

T4 is the storage form of thyroid, from which T3 is made. T4 is particularly important for brain functioning. Free T4 is the active form, and optimal range is 1–1.5. Most prescription thyroid is in the form of T4, including Synthroid and Levoxyl, or levothyroxine. Your body must remove one of the iodines from the T4 to become T3—the active form. Often, this conversion is not done well, and the FT3 will remain less than 3. Fatigue is almost always the result.

TSH is the most common thyroid lab that is drawn by every doctor across America. TSH, or thyroid-stimulating hormone, is released from the pituitary gland to tell your thyroid to make more hormone. If it is high, your thyroid is not working well and is not able to make adequate thyroid hormone. Normal levels will be read a 0.5–5; the American Academy of Endocrinology (the thyroid specialists) have stated the upper limit should be 3.0. That means, anything over 3 should be diagnosed as hypothyroidism. Of course, optimal levels of TSH are different: 1–1.5 is best.

Can you have a normal TSH and still have hypothyroidism? Yes! This is the most important fact to remember. If your doctor checks your TSH and says it's normal, there's nothing wrong with you, and the reason you're tired and overweight is that you're lazy. Find another doctor. Your TSH can be completely normal, even optimal, but still have a low thyroid.

Smoking can lower your TSH and can hide the fact that you have hypothyroidism or keep you undertreated.

There's also something called thyroid resistance. In this case, the thyroid gland and the pituitary are both functioning normally, but the receptor sites on each cell are defective. The thyroid is not binding as it should to the receptor site, and the hormone isn't getting inside the cell as it should. The most common cause is high stress and high cortisol levels. A high homocysteine can also cause this.

Often, patients will not respond to their thyroid medication when it's the synthetic levothyroixine or Synthroid, T4. In this case, a T3/T4 combination works much better. The two meds that I have found

117

to be much more effective in treating hypothyroidism are Armour Thyroid and Nature-Throid. These are a more bioidentical T3/T4 combo that will often allow you to have more energy and adequately treat lagging T3 levels.

Sometimes the T3/T4 in Armour Thyroid or Nature-Throid is not enough, and I'll have a compounding pharmacy make a T3/T4 med in the exact dosage needed.

Thyroid support is often needed, with supplements that contain iodine and selenium. Eating five brazil nuts a day has all the selenium the thyroid needs, and use iodized salt. Even some sea salts now have iodine added.

If your thyroid antibodies are high, a condition called Hashimoto's disease, then you are making antibodies to your thyroid and attacking the gland. This is the most common cause of hypothyroidism. Antibody levels should be less than 15. Anything over 15 is too high.

Hashimoto's, because it is an autoimmune disease, greatly increases your inflammation throughout your body. Because of this, it will increase your risk of breast cancer, earlier heart disease, and other autoimmune diseases such as rheumatoid arthritis. Therefore, it is important to try to reverse the antibodies and bring them down to as close to zero as possible.

First, you'll need to be on a gluten-free diet, as gluten is a common trigger of inflammation contributing to the disease. We'll discuss this more on the chapter on nutrition. Second, take a thyroid supplement with thyroid and adrenal extracts to help divert some of the antibodies to the extract and not your thyroid. Third, supplements to reduce overall inflammation are important. With this regimen, Hashimoto's can be reversed. It can take years, but it's worth the effort for your health.

The thyroid gland, like many parts of our body, diminishes its activity as we age, with fatigue being the number 1 complaint. There are some great books on thyroid disorders if you'd like a more comprehensive review. Two books I especially like is *Overcoming Thyroid Disorders* by Dr. Brownstein and *Stop the Thyroid Madness* by Janie A. Bowthorpe.

Chapter 16

Adrenal Fatigue

Work hard in silence, let your success be your noise.

—Frank Ocean

Robert was a long-haul truck driver with routes mainly up and down the West Coast. On a typical day, he would wake up at 6:00 AM and find it hard to get up and keep moving. He'd grab a quick breakfast, like a breakfast burrito or egg sandwich, washed down by four cups of coffee, and start moving.

He used to try to pack some healthier foods to snack on while driving, but now it was too much effort. His food consisted of fast food or truck stop food. His energy was lacking even more in the afternoon, and he relied on five-hour energy drinks to get through the day. The salt and sugar cravings were a daily struggle, and his belly seemed to grow larger day by day. Weight loss was next to impossible.

By 6:00 PM, he was calling it a night and parking the truck. Even though he was exhausted, his sleep was restless, and he never felt like he got a good night's sleep. The exhaustion made life a daily chore instead of a great adventure—the way he used to think about truck driving when he first started his career. Depression was now a way of life, and he had mental fatigue or brain fog. His doctor offered to start him on antidepressants, but after reading the side effects, he declined.

Does this sound familiar? If so, you may be suffering from adrenal fatigue.

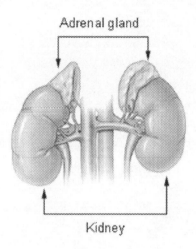

Adrenal gland

Kidney

The adrenal glands sit on top of the kidneys, and they produce over fifty hormones, with the major one being cortisol. Cortisol is the stress hormone. The levels of cortisol are high in the morning to get us going for the day and lowest at night so we can fall asleep more easily.

The adrenals deal with stress from everything that happens in your life, whether it's physical, mental, or emotional stress. They are responsible for the flight-or-fight response to stress. The problem is, many of us are faced with constant stress, whether it's from work or home, perhaps a physical illness, or even environmental toxins to which we're constantly exposed. What happens then is that the adrenal produces constant cortisol, and levels are too high. They can only keep this up for so long, and after a period, weeks to months, the cortisol levels begin to decline.

When cortisol levels are low, the symptoms are the following:

- Fatigue is the most common symptom. It's a constant tiredness that is always there, even in the morning, when you should feel rested. Often, you can feel a bit more energy in the evening and a second wind at around 11:00 PM, which makes sleep much more difficult;
- Poor memory or brain fog is very common. If you're trying to learn something new, it will take twice as long.
- Increased allergies.
- Cravings for foods that are high in salt, sugar, and fat.
- Autoimmune diseases.
- Weight gain, even when eating less calories.
- Poor muscle tone and decreased bone density.
- Low sex drive.
- Increased susceptibility to colds and flus and catching more than two colds a year.
- Cold hands and cold feet.
- Decreased ability to handle stress.
- Depression and anxiety.

Most doctors know nothing about adrenal fatigue, as this condition is not taught in medical school. The only accurate way to diagnose the condition is through salivary testing: a saliva sample is provided four times in one day—in the morning, at noon, around five, and before bedtime. This will show if there is a normal curve, where cortisol is high in the morning and lowest at night. (See pic.)

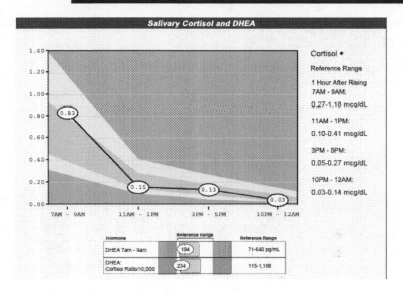

Normal Cortisol Curve

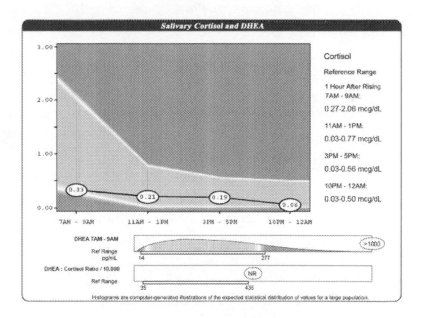

Adrenal Fatigue

Cortisol cannot be measured in the blood! Does any one of you like to have their blood drawn? No! Just the act of drawing blood, or coming at someone with a needle, is stressful and will bump up cortisol levels, giving an inaccurate result. Salivary testing, on the other hand, is painless and easy to complete at home.

The treatment for adrenal fatigue can be very successful and involves a number of natural supplements and specific dietary changes.

Treatment of adrenal fatigue are the following:

1. First of all, the adrenals store 95% of your vitamin C. Therefore, to be healthy, it is crucial that you have enough of this vitamin in your diet. It is best to get it in your food, which means plenty of fresh vegetables and fruit.

2. Diet is a huge factor in getting the adrenals to heal. The adrenals especially depend on protein to function. The high-carb diet that many of us eat is detrimental to this gland, and the first thing you're going to do is to start eating protein three times a day, especially for breakfast. Start off your day with a minimum of 15–20 g of protein. We'll go over this in much more detail in chapter. To get this much protein right off the bat, I typically will choose between three meals: a protein shake, two eggs and four pieces of bacon, or greek yogurt with nuts and berries.

3. If your adrenals are very low, liberally use the sea salts. Pink Himalayan sea salt or Celtic sea salt is the best. Here's a trick to get going in the morning. It sounds strange, but it works. Sprinkle some sea salt on the palm of your hand, and with no one watching, lick it off. When you coat the entire surface of the tongue with the sea salt, you'll get rapid absorption of the minerals. It's a pick-me-up for the adrenals.

4. There are supplements that are excellent for the health of the adrenals. Any supplement must include the B vitamins, zinc, and vitamin C. In addition, other nutrients are very useful, such as rhodiola, L-tyrosine, and chlorella. And there's something else called adrenal adaptogens, which is

desiccated adrenals, parotid, thymus, and spleen glandulars. I used to give patients six different bottles that contained all these ingredients, but I have found a product that has all of them in one capsule. It's much more convenient and cheaper! It's called Adrenal Manager, made by Xymogen. It's the most potent adrenal supplement I've found.

5. Sleep is critical for adrenal health. If you are not getting seven to nine hours of sleep per night, your adrenals cannot repair! And at least one morning per week, allow yourself to sleep in without guilt. Two mornings would be better, but at least get one morning where you give yourself permission to sleep as long as you'd like.

6. Improve nutrient absorption by drinking bone broth, greek yogurt, and fermented foods. Take a probiotic daily.

7. The other major hormone made by the adrenals is the DHEA. This is an antiaging hormone that naturally declines as we age. DHEA will help regulate cortisol levels, slow the aging process, help maintain muscle mass, and decrease abdominal fat.

8. Don't overtrain. If you are making yourself get up at 4:00 AM every day to go to the gym and then drag the rest of the day, you're not doing yourself any favors. This is contributing to low adrenal function and will make you sicker, not healthier. Pay attention to what your body is telling you, and treat it well.

9. Laugh and do something fun and enjoyable every day. You may only have ten to fifteen minutes to do this, but it's important. Find something to laugh about during your day, even if it's just something on the radio or a lame joke or a funny cat video on YouTube. And at the same time, be kind to yourself. Avoid saying anything negative about others and about yourself. Stay around positive people instead of those that want to drag you down with them.

Remember, our bodies are made to heal. And adrenal fatigue can heal. It won't happen overnight, as it can take from six months to two years, but the improvement in your symptoms once you have happy, healthy adrenals is well worth the steps to get there.

Chapter 17

DHEA, Pregnenolone, and Growth Hormone

The future belongs to those who believe in the beauty of their dreams.

—Eleanor Roosevelt

DHEA, or dehydroepiandrosterone, is made primarily in the adrenal glands. It is considered an antiaging hormone and is vital to maintain lean muscle mass.

Men make more of this hormone than women, and levels naturally start to decline at age thirty. It has so many amazing functions, which are the following:

1. Maintains lean muscle mass. When DHEA levels lower, we'll lose more muscle and gain more fat.
2. Enhances the immune system, making us more resistant to disease.
3. Decreases inflammation and reduces risk of autoimmune disease.

4. Reduces insulin levels, stimulates fat burning, and reduces risk of metabolic syndrome.
5. Improves libido and erectile dysfunction.
6. Protects against depression and improves mental functioning. Over age fifty, it helps to slow cognitive decline associated with aging and may help slow the progression of Alzheimer's and dementia.
7. Helps to protect against osteoporosis, as it increases bone density.

DHEA supplementation is generally not needed before age thirty. Dosages for men and women are different. On average, women need between 5 and 10 mg/day, and men need between 25 and 100 mg/day.

It's important to know that a portion of DHEA will convert to testosterone, and in women, this can cause side effects of acne, oily skin, and unwanted hair growth. Some women have higher levels of testosterone and cannot tolerate taking DHEA because of this. In this case, take a different type of DHEA called 7-keto DHEA. This type does not convert to testosterone, and it also has another beneficial effect of increasing fat metabolism. The dose of 7-keto DHEA is between 25 mg and 100 mg/day.

Levels of DHEA can be measured in the blood by measuring DHEA-S or sulfate. It can also be measured in the saliva and is included in most salivary panels.

Pregnenolone

This is the mothership hormone. It's made directly from cholesterol, and from it, all the sex hormones are made, including testosterone, estrogen, progesterone, and DHEA. It's primarily made in the adrenals, but other organs also make it, including even our retinas in the eyes, liver, salivary glands, testicles, ovaries, skin, and brain.

What are the functions of this hormone?

1) It's a natural anti-inflammatory. In large doses, it can reduce inflammation even from rheumatoid arthritis.
2) It protects our brain from dementia and is powerful at improving cognitive functioning. When you think of pregnenolone—and who doesn't at least three times a day?—think of brain booster and memory enhancer.
3) It makes people happier, reduces depression, and enhances feelings of well-being.
4) It improves the immune system.

Pregnenolone is made from cholesterol, and therefore, if your doctor is lowering your cholesterol with a statin drug, your production of hormones will decline, contributing to fatigue and muscle wasting.

The dose of pregnenolone is between 25 mg and 100 mg a day. It's best taken at night, as it may help with sleep and reduces inflammation while we slumber. However, in some, it can cause insomnia, so if it has this effect in you, take it in the morning.

Growth Hormone

How would you like to have one hormone that could increase your muscle mass, increase energy, decrease fat, improve sleep quality, improve libido and sexual performance, improve mood and cognition, reduce heart disease, and improve skin quality? Impossible, you say? No, not at all. Growth hormone, or the fountain-of-youth hormone, causes all these effects.

Produced in the pituitary gland, it helps regulate growth and metabolism and is highest when we're younger. It begins to decline at age twenty-five and decreases 15% every decade. (See pic.)

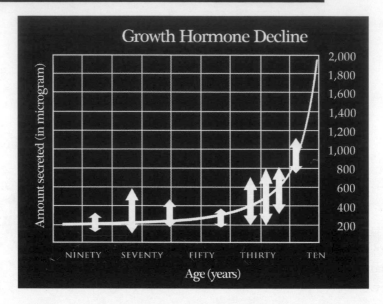

The secretion of growth hormone is highest at night while we sleep, so if we suffer from insomnia, we'll make less of it and age faster.

Once secreted by the pituitary, it is active in the blood for only a few minutes at a time, until it is converted by the liver into growth factors, the most active being one called IGF-1 (insulin-like growth factor). When we measure growth hormone, we actually measure levels of IGF-1.

Growth hormone cannot be taken as a pill, but rather, it must be administered as an injection you give yourself just before bedtime. Larger doses are given to increase muscle mass and reduce fat, and smaller doses are for general health and vitality.

Can it really do all it's proclaimed to do? Let's look at these effects more closely.

Increases fat loss. HGH improves the breakdown of fat, and patients who take HGH lose a greater percentage of fat with dietary changes. And the fat that's lost is often visceral fat, the deep fat that is so detrimental to our health. Now this doesn't mean that if you take growth hormone, you can eat whatever you want! You still have to change your diet to a higher-protein and lower-carb plan, but you'll find that you have greater fat loss.

Improves collagen production of skin. Have you noticed that as you age, your skin starts to sag? And wrinkle, of course. You can, in part, blame a declining level of HGH for this.

Strengthens immune system. As we age, we become more prone to disease as our immune system starts to fail. Without a healthy immunity, we are more at risk of developing infectious diseases such as colds, sinus infections and pneumonia, and cancer. Most people don't realize it, but one of the functions of the immune system is to find cells that are abnormal and kill them on the spot. If yours is lagging, it may not happen, and that abnormal cell becomes malignant.

Improves bone density. There are many reasons why our bones are so much stronger when we're young, but part of the reason is an abundance of growth hormone. With declining HGH, we lose bone density and muscle mass, putting us at greater risk of fractures. See people stooped over as they age? You can be sure they have osteoporosis or decreased bone density. (see pic)

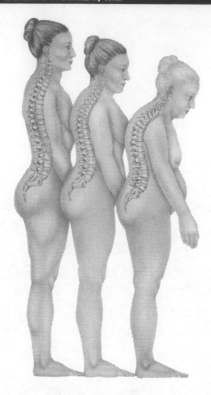

Regulates sleep patterns. Any of you over fifty may well know that as we age, our sleep pattern becomes more fragmented. Insomnia is the most common complaint I hear starting in middle age. There are so many reasons for this, and one of them is a lowering of HGH. Most people that start HGH will notice a normalized sleep pattern, and the sleep is deeper and more restorative.

If all this happens with this magical hormone, why don't we all take it, starting immediately? Well, like everything, there are a number of risks. It's important to realize that growth hormone is a controlled substance and can only be obtained with a prescription. It is not approved by the FDA for antiaging therapy. Of course, that doesn't always mean anything, as the FDA is in alliance with the pharmaceutical industry and is not always upright and honest about their purposes or doing what's best for society.

And the prescription is not cheap, running anywhere from $500 to $1500 a month. .

Theoretical risks to growth hormone include cancer. HGH causes growth, and potentially, if you already have a cancer, the hormone could cause it to grow more. However, other studies have shown a potential cancer-preventative effect from growth hormone. This makes sense when you consider that children who have the highest levels of HGH have very low rates of cancer. And our risk of cancer increases with aging, as our levels of growth hormone declines.

Other risks are carpal tunnel syndrome and insulin resistance.

Are there any alternatives to HGH or a natural way to increase our levels?

Yes, there is. A popular alternative to HGH is sermorelin or growth hormone–releasing hormone. It is the precursor of growth hormone and can allow our natural production of HGH to increase by stimulating the pituitary to make more. The advantages of sermorelin over HGH is cost—averaging $200 a month—and you can't overdose on growth hormone. Your body won't allow you to make too much of HGH with sermorelin. The effects are similar to HGH—more muscle mass, fat loss, increased energy, and more restful sleep.

There are two doses of sermorelin that are commonly used. Six-milligram injections are used for weight loss and antiaging properties, while two milligrams is used in body builders to bulk up their muscle mass.

You can order sermorelin from our website, and it comes in an easy-to-inject pen.

133

Section Three

NUTRITION

Chapter 18

Healthy Weight and BMI

Excuses don't get results.

Jimmy drives for a living and loves his work. He gets to spend almost every weekend home. A typical day starts early, at 6:00 AM after a restless night of sleep. In the morning, he's in a hurry, having no time for exercise, and breakfast consists of either a muffin or two donuts with a glass of orange juice or sometimes a breakfast burrito on the run. He'll chug down four cups of coffee by 10:00 AM, with nondairy, trans-fatty creamer and lots of sugar. Insulin has spiked since breakfast and has not been able to come down, with insulin resistance soon developing and diabetes in his future.

The stress of making the delivery in a timely manner makes cortisol levels rise, which causes more abdominal fat and damages the area of the brain called the hippocampus—the area responsible for short-term memory. Stress and coffee cause heartburn, so an antacid, the purple pill, is taken. This drug decreases the absorption of key nutrients such as B12, zinc, magnesium, and protein and thereby contributes to fatigue and more memory loss.

Lunch is a sandwich with turkey that has been injected with hormones, antibiotics, and saline on stale white bread with limp lettuce, or perhaps a mercury-laden tuna fish sandwich. Because he hears his wife's voice in his head telling him he's eating too much sugar, he gets a diet soda instead, which completely destroys his gut bacteria. And since he had a diet soda and not a regular one, he rationalizes he can have that dessert of an ice cream sandwich, ensuring that insulin will remain high.

Dinner is something similar but with french fries this time, which are fried in trans fats and oxidized, reheated oils, damaging every artery in the body. He dips them in ketchup that has high-fructose corn syrup, an ingredient that ruins the metabolism and increases appetite.

Once he parks the truck for the night, he's exhausted, mentally and physically, and puts off exercise just one more day. Collapsing in the cab of his truck, he watches a movie and binges on popcorn, making the insulin level skyrocket right before bedtime. He sleeps poorly again, keeping cortisol levels up, and insulin never really gets a chance to go down before he gets up in the morning to repeat the process all over again. Meanwhile, the high cortisol and insulin levels create havoc on the metabolism, causing more fat cells to form.

It likely is no surprise to any of you to know that obesity is the number 1 health problem of truckers and, indeed, of our society. Just look around and mentally count the number of people in the restaurant or at the grocery, school, or church; and see how many are overweight or obese versus how many are at an ideal weight. For long-haul truck drivers, 69% are obese. This is a crisis!

Why has it become such a problem? While there are many theories, much of it comes down to fast food, our love affair with carbs, inactivity, toxins, chemicals that disrupt our metabolism, and increasingly larger food portions have become the new norm.

If you compare the size of our plates in the 1950s versus now and even the size of a muffin then versus now, you'll see a huge difference. We have gotten used to eating more. (See pic.)

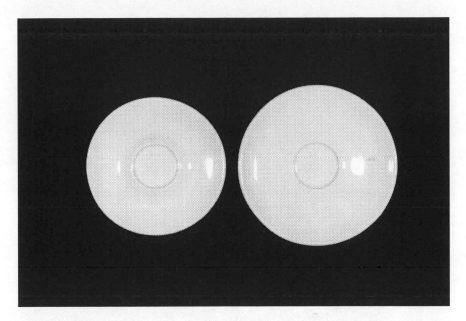

At the same time, we're cooking less and eating more fast food, which is about the same as eating chemicals. And food manufacturers have made the problem worse by adding more chemicals that make food taste better, increasing our desire and propensity to overeat. This includes MSG, high-fructose corn syrup, and gluten.

The problem in the trucking profession is eating on the run. And there's a direct correlation with the amount of time spent eating out and excess weight. This is especially true for fast food. There are so many calories in a fast food meal that one meal can contain the entire day's worth of calories! Eating fast food three times a week increases your risk of obesity by 33%. Truck stops aren't always better and offer a large range of unhealthy choices.

Another problem with truckers or anyone who drives a great deal is boredom. Boredom can lead to snacking, and endlessly snacking on salty, sweet foods mile after mile can pack on the calories in a hurry.

Of course, there's the inactivity, with long hours behind the wheel and tight deadlines to meet.

With the added weight comes added health risks, such as diabetes, high blood pressure, and sleep apnea, as discussed in the above chapters.

To determine if you're at a normal weight, overweight, or obese, we measure something called the BMI or body mass index. (See pic.)

HEIGHT ft/in	cm	90 / 41	100 / 45	110 / 50	120 / 54	130 / 59	140 / 64	150 / 68	160 / 73	170 / 77	180 / 82	190 / 86	200 / 91	210 / 95	220 / 100	230 / 104	240 / 109	250 / 113	260 / 118	270 / 122	280 / 127	290 / 132
4'8"	142.2	20	22	25	27	29	31	34	36	38	40	43	45	47	49	52	54	56	58	61	63	65
4'9"	144.7	19	22	24	26	28	30	32	35	37	39	41	43	45	48	50	52	54	56	58	61	63
4'10"	147.3	19	21	23	25	27	29	31	33	36	38	40	42	44	46	48	50	52	54	56	59	61
4'11"	149.8	18	20	22	24	26	28	30	32	34	36	38	40	42	44	46	48	51	53	55	57	59
4'12"	152.4	18	20	21	23	25	27	29	31	33	35	37	39	41	43	45	47	49	51	53	55	57
5'1"	154.9	17	19	21	23	25	26	28	30	32	34	36	38	40	42	43	45	47	49	51	53	55
5'2"	157.4	16	18	20	22	24	26	27	29	31	33	35	37	38	40	42	44	46	48	49	51	53
5'3"	160.0	16	18	19	21	23	25	27	28	30	32	34	35	37	39	41	43	44	46	48	50	51
5'4"	162.5	15	17	19	21	22	24	26	27	29	31	33	34	36	38	39	41	43	45	46	48	50
5'5"	165.1	15	17	18	20	22	23	25	27	28	30	32	33	35	37	38	40	42	43	45	47	48
5'6"	167.6	15	16	18	19	21	23	24	26	27	29	31	32	34	36	37	39	40	42	44	45	47
5'7"	170.1	14	16	17	19	20	22	24	25	27	28	30	31	33	34	36	38	39	41	42	44	45
5'8"	172.7	14	15	17	18	20	21	23	24	26	27	29	30	32	33	35	37	38	40	41	43	44
5'9"	175.2	13	15	16	18	19	21	22	24	25	27	28	30	31	33	34	35	37	38	40	41	43
5'10"	177.8	13	14	16	17	19	20	22	23	24	26	27	29	30	33	33	34	36	37	39	40	42
5'11"	180.3	13	14	15	17	18	20	21	22	24	25	27	28	29	31	32	33	35	36	38	39	40
5'12"	182.8	12	14	15	16	18	19	20	22	23	24	26	27	28	30	31	33	34	35	37	38	39
6'1"	185.4	12	13	15	16	17	18	20	21	22	24	25	26	28	29	30	32	33	34	36	37	38
6'2"	187.9	12	13	14	15	17	18	19	21	22	23	24	26	27	28	30	31	32	33	35	36	37
6'3"	190.5	11	13	14	15	16	18	19	20	21	23	24	25	26	28	29	30	31	33	34	35	36
6'4"	193.0	11	12	13	15	16	17	18	19	21	22	23	24	26	27	28	29	30	32	33	34	35
6'5"	195.5	11	12	13	14	15	17	18	19	20	21	23	24	25	26	27	28	30	31	32	33	34
6'6"	198.1	10	12	13	14	15	16	17	18	20	21	22	23	24	25	27	28	29	30	31	32	34
6'7"	200.6	10	11	12	14	15	16	17	18	19	20	21	23	24	25	26	27	28	29	30	32	33
6'8"	203.2	10	11	12	13	14	15	16	18	19	20	21	22	23	24	25	26	27	29	30	31	32
6'9"	205.7	10	11	12	13	14	15	16	17	18	19	20	21	23	24	25	26	27	28	29	30	31
6'10"	208.2	9	10	12	13	14	15	16	17	18	19	20	21	22	23	24	25	26	27	28	29	30
6'11"	210.8	9	10	11	12	13	14	15	16	17	18	19	20	21	22	23	25	26	27	28	29	30

Categories: Underweight | Healthy | Overweight | Obese | Extremely Obese

A BMI of less than 25 is normal; 25–29 is overweight; 30–39 is obese, and 40 or over is morbidly obese. BMI is not always accurate, as in body builders. In these cases, the BMI is always overestimated. The BMI can be underestimated in people that don't have a lot of muscle mass and only carry their weight around their abdomen. For both of these populations, a more accurate measurement of health is an abdominal waist circumference. A waist circumference of forty inches or more in men or thirty-five inches in women is an indicator of too much visceral fat, the dangerous, metabolically active type of fat.

An even simpler method of knowing if you have too much visceral fat is to simply lie down on your back and look at your belly. You should be able to see your ribs and a sloping down from there. If not, or if you can't even see your toes, there is too much fat.

As any of us that have tried dieting knows, weight comes on easily but comes off slowly. While this may seem discouraging, know that the weight will come off, one pound at a time. And with each pound of weight loss, there is a four-pound reduction in the joint load at our knees.

When you walk, the force on your knees is equivalent to 1½ times your body weight. This means that a two hundred-pound man will put three hundred pounds of pressure on his knees with each and every step! When going up and down stairs, the pressure is even greater. The force on each knee is two to three times your body weight.

While there is no easy "take the weight off quick" formula, there are some tricks of the trade that will allow the weight to come off more easily and consistently while increasing muscle mass. We'll discuss this in much detail in the upcoming chapters.

Chapter 19

COOKING ON THE ROAD

A goal should scare you a little and excite you a lot.

—Joe Vitale

Do you ever get tired of restaurant food? Food that's greasy, starchy, fried, fat, and sugar-laden with very little nutritional value? If not, then you've been eating this way for too long, and it's time to wake up your culinary senses. If so, then it's time to learn some simple methods of eating healthy food on the go, even when you're driving for twelve hours a day.

There are two things that every truck driver must have in their truck: (1) a Crock-Pot and (2) an electric skillet. With these two cooking utensils, a large variety of simple yet healthy and tasty meals can be made quickly and cheaply.

Another device that is very handy to have is a small blender. I use it to make protein shakes filled with frozen fruit and greens. It makes for a fast yet delicious and nutritious breakfast.

Also, an inverter is absolutely necessary if you don't have one built-in, as these appliances won't run off the power outlet from the truck.

Crock-Pot

With a Crock-Pot, you can make such a variety of meals that you don't have to eat the same thing twice in a month! Anything from soups to roast to enchiladas can be made. Get a small twelve-volt Crock-Pot with a lid that is strapped on. Amazon sells a great one for the road that plugs into your electric lighter. Check out RoadPro RPSL-350 12V 1.5 quart slow cooker. It's only big enough for one to two people, which is perfect for the truck. You can also purchase them at some truck stops. Then, to save on cleaning time, purchase slow cooker liners for the Crock-Pot. I get them on Amazon also. If you don't use the liners, make sure you use nonstick cooking spray to make cleanup easier.

Next, do your food preparation ahead of time by chopping up your vegetable and placing them in ziplock bags in your refrigerator. You can also purchase canned vegetables and beans, but realize that most canned food does not have as much nutrition as fresh.

There is such a variety of recipes online and in cookbooks for breakfast, lunch, and dinner. Take some time and research what sounds good to you. I like to stick to a lower carb count, which means no potatoes, but if your weight is not a problem, you can add a potato if you like.

You'll want to keep some basic seasonings in the truck, with the mainstays being sea salt, pepper, garlic powder, Italian seasoning, chili powder, cumin, and Lawry's seasoned salt. The most nutritious sea salt is Himalayan sea salt, the pink stuff. Celtic sea salt is also very good. Both are loaded with minerals that are good for the body. If you have another favorite spice, by all means, include it in your mix. See chapter 21 for some great recipes, and start collecting your favorites.

The other indispensable cooking utensil for the long-haul trucker is an electric skillet. With one skillet, an almost endless variety of food can be made—everything from stir-fry to eggs and bacon to pancakes. You can easily make hamburgers. Buy the frozen, 100% premade burgers at Costco to keep it really simple. Add salt and pepper, a little BBQ sauce if you like, some cheese; and there you go!

Use your skillet to try other recipes, such as stir-fry. Take either a chicken or steak; cut into strips; and add in your favorite vegetables, such as bell pepper, onions, carrots, and broccoli. Then stir-fry in sesame, coconut, or avocado oil; and combine it with soy sauce, brown sugar, and cornstarch.

Eat the stir-fry without rice, as rice is very high in carbs, has little nutritional value, and is often high in arsenic.

Again, plan ahead and make weekly stops at Walmart or any grocery store along the way to stock up on needed supplies. And if you ever get a chance to visit a farmers' market, you'll find your most nutritious and best-tasting produce there.

A refrigerator is also a must, and there are a number of refrigerators available online. The best one for you will depend on if you're a short- or long-haul trucker and how much room there is in the truck. Sometimes a cooler is all you need if you're only gone for a night or two.

Healthy snacks are also important. Who doesn't get bored traveling for miles on end? And with boredom comes snacking. Just remember, those calories count and add up fast. Look at these ideas for low-carb, healthy snacks you can take on the road.

Sunflower seeds. These are nutritious and delicious. Make sure you're getting the seeds still in the shells, as that will dramatically slow down the consumption.

Beef jerky. Purchase only ones without MSG, added nitrites, or sugar. MSG is a chemical that is used to enhance flavor but also causes increased appetite, headaches, sweating, and flushing. MSG overstimulates our nervous system, and the effects are cumulative with continued exposure.

Beef jerky brands without MSG and that are low in sugar are

- Steve's PaleoGoods,
- Country Archer,
- Biltong,
- Think Jerky,
- Oberto,
- Old Wisconsin,
- People's Choice, and
- Naked Cow.

You can find any of these on Amazon.

Nuts. Nuts are highly nutritious, moderately high in protein, and low in carbs. Nuts have different amounts of carbs, and the best nuts are the lowest in carbs. The following are the carb contents of nuts:

- Pecans, macadamia nuts, and brazil nuts—4
- Hazelnuts, walnuts, and peanuts—7
- Almonds—10
- Pistachios—18
- Cashews—27

So as you can see, cashews contain a large amount of carbs, and if you're trying to lose weight on a low-carb diet, they should be avoided. Eat pecans, macadamia nuts, and brazil nuts. These can be eaten more freely.

- Boiled eggs. These are easy, with zero carbs.
- Cheese. These have zero carbs.

- Guacamole. Buy the individual packets. You can purchase these at Costco. Use celery and carrot sticks to dip, not chips!
- Hummus. This is another great dip for your vegetables. These are low in carbs and delicious.
- Meat and cheese rolls. Be creative and use meat slices as your wrap. Inside I like to add a cheese stick, bell peppers, pickles, and spinach; but add whatever vegetables and fillings you'd like. Just keep it low carb—no potatoes or bread!
- Cucumber boats filled with tuna salad.
- Celery with almond butter.
- Tomato slices topped with mozzarella cheese and basil, with a little balsamic vinegar drizzled over all.
- Dill pickles or sugar-free sweet pickles.
- Avocado.
- Berries. These are lower in carbs than other fruits and are so good for you.
- Premier or Atkins protein drinks. Both brands are low in sugar and carbs and high in protein. Keep some stocked in your refrigerator for a quick breakfast or snack.

There are many other low-carb recipes and snacks. I'm just giving you an idea of how to start. Cater it to your own tastes and needs while keeping the carb count down.

What if you just don't feel like cooking today and you want to grab something on the run? In the next chapter, we'll talk about healthy restaurant choices and what to avoid.

Chapter 20

HEALTHY RESTAURANT CHOICES

The secret of getting ahead is getting started.

—Mark Twain.

Eating on the run often leads to unhealthy choices. There are so many foods that are high in sugar, fried in rancid trans fat, have no nutritional value, and are highly inflammatory. The healthy trucker has to learn what she or he can or cannot eat.

Let's look at a typical meal at the truck stop.

Soggy chicken fingers, french fries cooked ten hours ago, limp sandwiches made a week ago, hot dogs dripping in grease that quickly lines your arteries with plaque, and fruit that is weeks old and has lost its vitamins.

Can a body live on that? No! All it does is create more inflammation and more fat, leaving you feeling tired with brain fog and cravings to eat more of the crap two hours later.

We can't continue to feed our bodies in this way if we expect them to function like a well-oiled and well-tuned machine.

There is very little meal choices at a truck stop that are good for your body and soul. If you can find a chef's salad where the meat hasn't spoiled and the lettuce isn't too wilted, that's great. Don't use ranch or other high in sugar/fat/carb dressings, but keep some balsamic vinegar or low-carb Italian dressings in your truck. Sprinkle some sunflower seeds on top or add some shredded cheese.

There are some truck stops with great reputations, and I'm sure that as you read this, you'll be able to add more. A few of them include the following:

- Iowa 80 Truckstop at 755 W., Iowa 80 Road, Walcott, Iowa, 52773. This is the largest truck stop in the world, with a hundred thousand-square-feet complex, featuring a theater, dentist's office, chiropractor, and a great salad bar. The food is made fresh. And it includes many tempting bakery desserts, but just say no to those.
- Morris Travel Center at 21 Romines Dr., Morris, IL, 60450. They have several restaurants with great salads, salmon, and fresh foods.
- Florida 595 Truck Stop at Intersection of I-595 and 441. They have a home-style diner and fresh food, and they offer online deals for many different services.
- Bosselman Travel Center at Grand Island, NE, I-80, exit 312. This caters to truckers, is clean, and has a variety of eating choices, including Subway.

Fast food has a bad reputation, which is well-earned. But there are more fast food restaurants now that have food choices that are nutritious and healthy. The best fast food that's healthy can be found at the following:

- *Subway.* Get their salad with chicken breast and loads of veggies.

- *Chipotle.* Limit the rice and no chips, but load up on meat, beans, and veggies.
- *Panera Bread.* Any of the salads are great, but leave out the bread.
- *Chick-fil-A.* Get the grilled chicken cool wrap or grilled chicken nuggets, with a superfood salad.
- *Arby's.* Their roast turkey farmhouse salad with Italian lite dressing is delicious.
- *Carl's Jr.* Their low-carb cheeseburger is basically a hamburger wrapped in lettuce instead of a bun.
- *KFC.* Get the grilled chicken with green beans. Keep it low carb.
- *Panda Express.* Get the broccoli beef with a side of veggies. Skip the rice and noodles.
- *McDonald's.* Get the grilled, honey-roasted chicken snack wrap or premium chicken salad with low-fat balsamic vinaigrette dressing. If you can't walk into a McDonald's without coming out with fries, don't go in!
- *Wendy's.* Get the salads with chicken, veggies, and berries.

There are many other restaurants out there, of course. Just choose the grilled meats over fried, and get a salad whenever you can. And choose water to drink. You don't need sugar and chemical-laden sodas. I like water with a little flavor, even a splash of lemon or lime. The lemon is a great detoxifier and helps keep you more alkaline. Drink it throughout the day.

However you decide to refuel your body, in the next chapter, I'm going to tell you about a way to cook for yourself with prep, grocery shopping, cutting, or peeling and how to carry meats for months at a time without spoiling.

Chapter 21

THRIVE

Ken is a long-haul truck driver who is gone for weeks at a time. After putting on twenty pounds in the first six months of work, he decided some changes had to be made and quickly, before things got out of hand. The first order of business was preparing meals for himself, ones that were nutritious, low in starch and carbs, and high in flavor. However, the thought of planning meals, shopping for ingredients weekly, washing, chopping, storing the produce, and making room in the tiny freezer for meat was a daunting task for him. Until he discovered Thrive.

Thrive is a company that sells many non-GMO foods that have been dehydrated, freeze-dried, and most are able to be stored for years unopened without refrigeration. The Thrive foods consists of the same foods you would buy at the market, such as fruit, veggies, grains, meat, and dairy. Using flash-freeze technology, the foods retain 99% of the nutrients, color, and texture of foods. In fact, the vegetables and fruit are often higher in vitamins than the produce found at the grocery because as soon as the ripened fruit is picked, it is washed, sliced, and dehydrated and freeze-dried.

Compare this to the produce found in supermarkets. Some veggies, like lettuce or spinach, might have been picked just two to three weeks ago. Other produce, such as apples, can sit in cold storage for an entire year before being sold! In fact, in one study, the average apple sold in a grocery store is fourteen months old. Why is this a problem? Nutrients and vitamins. Apples are known to be high in antioxidants called polyphenols. They help fight cancer, decrease inflammation, and help reduce fatigue after exercise. But as soon as an apple is picked, it begins to lose these vital nutrients, and one that's been stored for a year has none remaining. Zero.

This is true for most vegetables and fruits. The longer they sit on the shelf, the lower the nutrients. The best produce is, therefore, found in what you grow that can be eaten right after picking or at the farmers' market, which sells only locally grown, fresh produce.

However, for the trucker, this is the problem. You can't grow a garden in the bed of your truck, and it's mighty inconvenient to hunt down all the local farmers' markets!

Instead, to overcome this problem, we use Thrive. It's the next best thing to the fruit that is just picked from the tree. The company allows the fruit or vegetable to ripen, then they're picked. This is again unlike many other fruits that are picked before ripening and, therefore, never have the amount of nutrients it should or could have.

Almost 52% of vitamin C in green beans is lost after two days. Thrive blueberries contain 40% more calcium than frozen; six times more vitamin A in spinach than store-bought; and twenty-one times more vitamin C in peaches than store-bought.

The products also contain no MSG, hydrogenated oils, preservatives, or artificial flavors and colors, and use non-GMO whenever possible. They won't accept sources from China or anywhere else that may be of poor quality. They use dozens of sources that are regulated by and conform to FDA and USDA requirements.

But the best thing I love about Thrive is the ease of use. It makes cooking and preparing a snap!

You simply purchase online the meat, fruit, and vegetables you want. I also get cheese, milk, spices, and a wonderful snack the kids love called yogurt bites. Everything is already cleaned and diced, so you open the can you want to use and pour it in. This way, meat can be carried in your truck in cans that do not require refrigeration, freezing, or thawing; and it is ready to use.

There are some drawbacks. You can't cook a fresh hamburger patty or fry up some bacon slices, for example. But for casseroles, Crock-Pot, and stir-fry, there is nothing easier.

The fruit is so good that my kids will eat an entire large can of peaches or strawberries in one sitting if I don't catch them. I love eating the green beans and asparagus right out of the jar without cooking. I'll throw the kale into my smoothies in the morning. I have to disguise kale, or my husband would never eat it.

Another advantage to using Thrive is that it solves the problem of wasting food. No longer will you have to throw out fruit or veggies that have gone bad or started to mold and wilt. This is a huge savings in the long run! Americans throw out an average of 25–60% of their food, and most of it comes from food that has spoiled. That's an average of $2000 to $4000 per year.

In the chapter on recipes, I'll have some Thrive recipes that you can use, and many more are online. There's also a Thrive cookbook that is helpful. To sign up for Thrive, go to ThriveLife.com/HealthyLiving.

Chapter 22

Recipes

Discovery consists of looking at the same thing as everyone else and thinking something different.

Recipes
Simple Crock-Pot Recipes

Beef Stew
1 package of beef stew meat
1 carrot, sliced
1 can of green beans
1 small onion, diced

Seasoned salt, pepper, and garlic to taste
Place beef stew meat at bottom of Crock-Pot. Add your onion on top then carrots and green beans. Sprinkle with spices. Cover and cook on low for 8 hrs.

Chicken Tortilla Soup

1 chicken breast, cut into chunks or 1 12-oz. can of canned chicken chunks
1 packet of taco seasoning
1 jar of salsa
1 32-oz. chicken broth
1 can of black beans
½ onion, diced

Some bell peppers if you like
Place the chicken at the bottom of the crock then the onions (and bell peppers if you want), then sprinkle with taco seasoning meat. Open can of salsa and pour on top. Pour can of chicken broth over all. Drain can of beans, then pour beans on top of everything. Cook on low for 8–10 hrs. or high for 6 hrs. Thirty minutes before it's ready, pull out the chicken and shred, then place back in the pot for another 30 mins. This is so yummy. Enjoy!

Spaghetti and Meatballs

1-lb. frozen meatballs
1 28-oz. jar of spaghetti sauce of your choice (like Ragú or Prego)
12-oz. dry spaghetti
½ the jar sauce of water

Place spaghetti noodles on bottom of crock. Pour sauce and water over noodles. Place meatballs on top and stir. Add a tablespoon of olive oil if you like, for flavor and to keep noodles from sticking. Cook on low for 5–6 hrs.

Shredded Pork Roast

2 slices of bacon
1-lb. butt roast
2 3 garlic cloves
Sea salt

Line the crock with slices of bacon. Cut some slits into the roast, and place garlic cloves. Sprinkle with sea salt. Place on top of bacon, skin side up. Cook on low for 8–10 hrs. Check it after 8. Shred it with forks and enjoy!

Roast Vegetables

1 red bell pepper
1 sweet potato
1 carrot
1 small zucchini
Olive oil
Seasonings of your choice—Italian is great and seasoned salt and pepper

Cut all the above in slices. Spray Crock-Pot with cooking spray, place all vegetables in the pot. Season as desired, and add 1 tbsp. of olive oil. Cook on low 4–6 hrs., and stir midway.

Chicken Chili

1 chicken breast
1 can of chicken broth
1 can of great northern beans, drained
½ cup of salsa verde
Seasoned salt, chili powder, and garlic powder
Optional toppings (cilantro, sour cream, shredded cheese, green onions, and olives)

Place chicken breast on bottom of crock. Pour broth over top and add beans and salsa verde. Sprinkle with seasonings, including ½–1 tsp. of chili powder and a dash of garlic powder. Cook on low for 6–8 hrs., until chicken is easily shred with a fork. Serve with desired toppings.

Ravioli

1½ cups of ravioli of your choice
1 16-oz. jar spaghetti sauce
1 cup of mozzarella cheese

Spray pot with cooking spray. Pour small amount of sauce on the bottom. Layer with ravioli, sauce, and cheese. Continue layers until it's ¾ full to the top. Cook on low for 3–4 hrs.

Turkey Crock-Pot

1-lb. boneless turkey breast (or 1½–2 with bone)
½ of a 16-oz. can of cranberry sauce
½ envelope of dry onion soup mix

Put turkey on bottom of crock, then put cranberry sauce on top. Sprinkle about ½ of the envelope of onion soup mix on top. Cook on high for 2 hrs. Then reduce heat to low, and cook for another 2–4 hrs.

Pork Chops

2 pork chops
½ envelope of dry onion soup mix
1 10-oz. can of chicken broth

If you'd like to brown the pork chops first, you can, but it's not essential. Place them on the bottom of the crock. Mix the soup mix and chicken broth in a bowl, then pour it over the top. Cook on low heat for 6–8 hrs.

Spicy Black-Eyed Peas

½ lb. of dried black-eyed peas, sorted and rinsed
3 cups of water
½ onion, diced
1 clove of garlic
½ red bell pepper
4-oz. diced ham
2 slices of bacon
Salt and pepper to taste
½ tsp. of cumin
1 chicken bouillon cube

Pour water into Crock-Pot, add bouillon cube, and dissolve. Combine and add all other ingredients. Cook on low for 6–8 hrs. or until beans are tender.

There are so many other recipes you can find on the internet. Be creative, and plan ahead. When you're finally at home for a few days, take a little time to plan your meals for the next trip, whether it's only for a few days or a few weeks. It does take some planning, but the results are so worth the effort. You'll find that you are saving money too.

Snack Recipes
These will need to be made at home before hitting the road again.

Almond Donuts

1 cup of almond meal
4 tbsp. of honey
2 large eggs
¼ tsp. of baking soda
2 tsp. of vanilla

Preheat oven to 300F. Grease the donut pan. Mix ingredients in large mixing bowl until smooth. Fill ½ of each donut cavity. Bake for 10–15 mins. until a toothpick comes out clean. Do not overbake! Allow to cool before removing the donuts. These will last for 3–4 days, longer in the refrigerator. Eat as is or apply a topping, such as almond butter or sugar-free jam.

No-Crust Pizza

This is a great recipe and can be made ahead of your trip.
Take mozzarella shredded cheese, place on skillet in a 10-inch circle over medium heat. When the cheese starts to bubble, add toppings. I like pepperoni, mushrooms, and olives. Once the edges are brown all around, slide onto plate. Let cool so you can cut them into pizza slices, and enjoy!

Blueberry Nutty Cereal

2 cups of pecans, chopped
1/3 cup of coconut oil
6 medium dates, pitted
1 cup of pumpkin seeds
1 tbsp. of vanilla
2 tsp. of cinnamon
½ tsp. of sea salt
½ cup of coconut flakes, unsweetened
½ cup of dried blueberries

Preheat oven to 325°F. Put half the pecans, coconut oil, and dates in a food processor. Pulse until finely ground. Add the remainder of pecans and pumpkin seeds, and pulse just once or twice to rough chop. Transfer to a bowl, and add vanilla, cinnamon, and salt. Stir and spread on baking sheet. Bake for 20 mins. until browned. Remove, let cool, and stir in the coconut and blueberries. Store in airtight container. This makes a delicious substitute for cereal and is a nutritious snack!

Nut and Fruit Yummies

2 cups of the nuts of choice—almonds, pecans, walnuts, macadamia nuts, chopped
2 tbsp. sunflower seeds
¼ cup of dried cranberries
¼ cup of raisins
¼ cup of dried apricots
½ tsp. of sea salt, coarse
2 large egg whites

Preheat oven to 350°F. Combine all ingredients in a large bowl. Line a baking sheet with parchment paper and drop the mix in even spoonfuls, 2 tbsp. each. Bake for 10 mins. until the nuts are lightly roasted. Cool completely. Store in airtight container.

Thrive Recipes

Southwest Chicken Fajitas

2 tbsp. butter
1 tbsp. minced garlic
¾ cup of Thrive onion slices
¾ cup of Thrive red bell peppers
2 cups of water
1½ cups of Thrive seasoned chicken slices
3 tbsp. of Thrive green chili peppers
½ tsp. of cumin
½ tsp. of chili powder
½ tsp. of Thrive chef's choice seasoning
1 tbsp. Thrive velouté chicken gravy
1 tsp. of lime juice

Corn tortillas, 4 in.
½ cup of shredded cheddar cheese

Cilantro, for topping if desired
Sauté garlic in butter. Add onion slices, bell peppers, and chicken slices; and toast lightly. Add in remaining ingredients except velouté and lime juice. Simmer until water is mostly reduced. Sprinkle in velouté while stirring, and then finish with the lime juice. Mix should be slightly saucy. Allow to cook for another minute, and serve with tortillas and toppings.

Southwest Queso Dip

2 slices of bacon, diced
1 tbsp. garlic, minced
1½ cups of water
1 tbsp. of Thrive red bell peppers
1 tbsp. of Thrive onion slices
1 tbsp. of Thrive sweet corn
2 tbsp. of Thrive green chili peppers
3 tbsp. of Thrive velouté chicken gravy
½ tsp. of Thrive chef's choice seasoning
¼ tsp. of cumin
½ tsp. of chili powder
2 tsp. of hot sauce, if desired
¼ cup of milk
2 cups of shredded cheddar cheese

Vegetables for dipping
In a small saucepan, cook bacon until crispy. Drain half the fat, and add in the garlic. Sauté until lightly brown. Add remaining ingredients except the milk and cheese. Simmer for 3 mins. or until slightly thick. Add in milk and cheese and remove from heat. Stir until smooth. Serve with fresh veggies for dipping.

Thrive in a Jar

The following recipes are simple to make and can be put together at home before you leave. Then each night for dinner, you simply choose which dinner you want since most of the prep has already been done! Normally, I make these in a mason jar, but for truckers, it may be best to put them in a ziplock bag that can then be thrown away after use. This will decrease the need for storage of glass bottles. You can also use a vacuum sealer, which will allow the food to stay preserved for longer. If vacuum sealing, be sure that all powders, seasonings, and smaller items are put into the pouch first and are the furthest away from where the vacuum will be sucking the air out so that the powders, seasonings, etc. remain in the pouch.

Using ziplock bags will work for short periods, up to three weeks at a time, so long as they don't pick up moisture and aren't exposed to temperatures above 75°F or light for prolonged periods. Temperatures above 75°F and exposure to light and moisture will degrade the food.

Spaghetti
Layer the following in a bag or vacuum sealer:

½ cup of Thrive ground beef
1 cup of Thrive tomato sauce
2 tsp. of garlic powder
2 tsp. of Thrive chef's choice seasoning
2 tbsp. of Thrive Italian seasoning
¼ cup of Thrive sausage crumbles
½ cup of Thrive zucchini
¼ cup of Thrive chopped onions
¼ cup of Thrive chopped celery
½ cup of Thrive mushrooms
½ cup of Thrive tomato dices

Boil 5 cups of water. Add contents of bag and stir until well blended. Simmer for 10–15 mins. until veggies and meat are fully rehydrated. Add more water if needed. Serve over pasta, or if low carb, serve in a bowl with shredded mozzarella cheese on top.

Cheesy Sausage Frittata

½ cup of Thrive scrambled egg mix
½ cup of Thrive sausage crumbles
½ cup of Thrive vegetables of choice (onions, bell pepper, mushrooms, green beans, for example)
½ cup of Thrive cheddar cheese
2 tsp. of chives
1 tsp. of Thrive onions, diced
½ tsp. of Thrive chef's choice seasoning

Pour all the ingredients in a bowl, and place 1½ cups of water over all. Stir and mix ingredients. Let it stand for a few minutes to allow for rehydration. Heat skillet. Add egg mixture to pan, and cook for 20 mins. or until eggs are firmly set. Top should be lightly browned and pulled from edges slightly.

Chicken Broccoli Stir-Fry Jar Meal

1 cup of Thrive chicken pieces
¼ cup of chicken bouillon
3 tbsp. of cornstarch
2 tbsp. of sugar
2 tsp. of dried parsley
½ tsp. of ground ginger
¼ tsp. of crushed, dried red pepper flakes
1 cup of Thrive dried broccoli
¼ cup of Thrive carrots, diced
4 tbsp. of Thrive chopped onions
½ cup of Thrive green peppers

1 cup of Thrive instant rice

Layer ingredients in a ziploc bag. Add 4 cups of water to a skillet and bring to boil. Add mix, and stir well. Turn off heat, and let it rest for 10 mins. After your rest period, simmer for 20–25 mins. while covered.

Home-Style Beef Stew

1 cup of Thrive beef dices
½ cup of Thrive green beans
½ cup of Thrive corn
½ cup of tomato dices
¼ cup of Thrive peas
¼ cup of Thrive celery
¼ cup of Thrive carrots
2 tbsp. of Thrive instant red beans
2 tbsp. of Thrive tomato powder
1½ tbsp. of instant beef bouillon
2 tbsp. of Thrive minced onions
1 tsp. of Lawry's seasoned salt
2 tsp. of cornstarch
Dash of pepper

Add contents to 8 cups of hot water. Simmer for 20 mins. This serves 4 people or 1 with leftovers.

Taco Soup

1 cup of Thrive sausage crumbles
¾ cup of Thrive ground beef
¼ cup of Thrive chopped onions
1 cup of Thrive instant black beans
1/3 cup of Thrive corn
4 tbsp. of mixed bell peppers

2–3 tbsp. of Thrive green chilis
3 tbsp. of taco seasoning mix
1–2 tbsp. of cumin
¼ cup of Thrive sour cream powder
¼ cup of Thrive tomato powder
¼ cup of Thrive cheddar cheese
1 tbsp. of Thrive cilantro

Add all ingredients to a large pot. Mix with 7 cups of water. Bring to a boil, and simmer for 15–20 minutes. You can easily half the recipe if desired.

Hearty Vegetable Soup

2 tsp. of chicken bouillon
¼ cup of Thrive broccoli
¼ cup of Thrive carrots
¼ cup of Thrive zucchini
1/8 cup of Thrive green onions
¼ cup of Thrive green peas
½ cup of Thrive corn
¼ cup of Thrive asparagus
1/8 cup of Thrive diced onions
½ cup of Thrive green beans
1/8 cup of Thrive mixed red and green peppers
¼ cups of Thrive red bell pepper chunks
1 tsp. of chef's choice seasoning
½ cup of Thrive shredded cheddar cheese

To make, add all ingredients to 4 cups of water in a pot. Cook over medium heat until boiling; simmer for 15 mins.

Chicken Potpie

1 cup of Thrive chicken dices
1/3 cup of Thrive carrot dices
½ cup of Thrive chopped onions
½ cup of Thrive potato dices
1/3 cup of Thrive green peas
1/3 cup of Thrive velouté gravy
1 tbsp. of Thrive butter powder
½ tbsp. of Thrive nonfat powdered milk
1 tbsp. of ground sage
½ tsp. of black pepper
1 tbsp. of dried parsley
½ tsp. of Lawry's seasoned salt

Add contents to 6 cups of water, and bring to a boil. Simmer 10–15 mins. If desired, you may add a tablespoon of flour to thicken.

Corn Spicy Salsa

2 tbsp. of Thrive diced onions
½ cup of Thrive corn
¼ cup of Thrive green bell peppers
2 tbsp. of Thrive green chili peppers
2 tbsp. of Thrive cilantro
½ tbsp. of Thrive chef's choice seasoning
2 cups of Thrive tomato dices
1 tsp. of Thrive summer limeade
½ tsp. of salt
1 tbsp. of Cholula hot sauce
1¼ cup of water

Add all ingredients in a bowl. Stir to mix. Refrigerate for 1 hour to enhance flavors. This is delicious and can be eaten as a fresh vegetable without chips!

Chicken Fajitas

1½ cups of thrive chicken slices
¾ cup of Thrive onion slices
½ cup of Thrive green chili peppers
½ cup of Thrive green bell peppers
¾ cup of Thrive red bell peppers
½ tsp. of chili powder
½ tsp. of cumin
½ tsp. of chicken bouillon
½ tsp. of chef's choice seasoning
½ tsp. of Thrive cilantro
¼ tsp. of garlic powder
1/8 tsp. of Thrive summer limeade

Add all ingredients to 2 cups of warm water, and let it sit for 8 mins. Drain off excess water. Add 1–2 tbsp. of avocado oil to skillet and heat until hot. Add chicken mixture, and stir until lightly browned. Serve with cheese, corn salsa, and guacamole if desired.

Chicken Noodle Soup

1 cup of Thrive chicken
1/3 cup of Thrive onion
1½ cups of favorite Thrive veggies
¼ cup of thrive carrots
½ cup of Thrive béchamel sauce powder
2/3 cup of Thrive velouté sauce powder
1 tbsp. of chicken bouillon

Place in pot, and add 8 cups water. Simmer for 5 mins. Add noodles and simmer 10 more minutes.

Chicken Salad

1 tsp. of Thrive salad seasoning
1/8 cup of Thrive celery
1 cup of Thrive chicken, diced
1 tbsp. of Thrive diced onions
1/8 cup of Thrive cranberries
¼ cup of Thrive apples, diced

Add ¾ cup plus 1 tbsp. cold water. Let it sit for 10 mins. Add 1 tbsp. of mayo if desired. Eat with fresh veggies, bread, or crackers.

Spicy, Low-Carb Roasted Veggie Snack Mix

1 cup of Thrive asparagus
1 cup of Thrive cauliflower
1 cup of Thrive red bell peppers
1 cup of Thrive zucchini
1 cup of Thrive onion slices
1 cup of tomato dices
½ cup of Thrive green chilies
½ cup of Thrive sausage crumbles
½ cup of Thrive cheddar cheese
1/3–½ cup of melted coconut oil
1 tsp. of Thrive garlic
1 tsp. of Bolner's Fiesta Brand extra fancy taco seasoning or seasoning of your choice.

In a large pan or cookie sheet, gently mix together all the vegetables. In a saucepan, gently heat the coconut oil, minced garlic, and seasoning until the garlic is cooked. Drizzle over the veggies while gently stirring. Bake at 250°F for 12–18 mins., stirring every 3 mins. Watch and stir closely to prevent over toasting. After removing from the oven, add dry sausage crumbles and cheddar cheese. Store in closed container.

Creamy Sausage Zuppa Toscana

3/8 cup of Thrive potato chunks
2 tbsp. of Thrive bechamel creamy white sauce
3/8 cup of Thrive sour cream powder
3/8 cup of Thrive mashed potatoes, or for lower carb, grind Thrive cauliflower into powder and use 1/3 cup
½ tbsp. of Thrive chicken bouillon
¼ tsp. of Thrive chef's choice seasoning
1/8 tsp. of crushed red pepper flakes
¼ tsp. of garlic powder
3/8 cup of Thrive chopped spinach
2 tbsp. of Thrive chopped onions
3/8 cup of Thrive sausage crumbles

Place all ingredients in a mason jar or ziplock bag. When ready to use, dump contents of the jar into a pot with 2½ cups of cold water. Stir ingredients into water until all lumps are gone. Bring to a boil, turn down to medium heat, and let simmer for about 10–15 mins. or until potatoes and sausage are soft.

Gazpacho

¾ cup of fresh cucumber, peeled and small diced
½ tsp. of Thrive summer limeade
¼ cup of Thrive chopped onions
¾ cup of tomato dices
2 tbsp. of Thrive green chili peppers
¼ cup of Thrive tomato powder
½ tsp. of Thrive garlic
¾ tsp. of Thrive chef's choice
2 cups of cold water
¼ tsp. of salt
1 tbsp. of Cholula or other hot sauce
1 tbsp. of Thrive cilantro

Mix all ingredients and chill for 30 mins.

Section Four

ALTERNATIVE MEDICINE

Chapter 23

MiraDry

Act the way you'd like to be and soon you'll be the way you act.

—Leonard Cohen.

If you are working on something you really care about, you don't have to be pushed. The vision pulls you.

—Steve Jobs

Sweating is natural. Our body sweats to cool itself off and to detoxify. Most of us don't release it, but the skin is the largest organ in the body and is vital for detoxification. We have between two and four million sweat glands throughout our body, but the ones we're most concerned about are the ones in the underarms.

Only 2% of our sweat glands are in the underarms, yet they are the most embarrassing, leading to obvious sweat marks and body odor. We use antiperspirants and deodorants, which contain aluminum chloride that reduce sweating by only 20%. Deodorants don't reduce sweating, but they reduce odor. Antiperspirants won't reduce odor, but they reduce sweating.

There is concern about the aluminum in the antiperspirants, as it is a toxic metal that is absorbed through the skin. Aluminum has been implicated in Alzheimer's, dementia, breast cancer, and autoimmune diseases.

For 3% of the population, the combination of antiperspirants and deodorants are not effective. Called hyperhidrosis, excessive sweating can occur in the underarms (or axilla), hands, or feet. Axillary sweating is the most embarrassing, leaving sweat stains and causing body odor that is obvious to anyone around. Even prescription antiperspirants won't work, and they often lead to skin irritation.

Patients with this condition will often only wear black and put Kleenex, gauze, and even maxi pads under their arms to try to hide the sweating.

Until now, Botox has been the only effective treatment for hyperhidrosis. Botox injections are done under the arms and block the chemical that activates the sweat glands. The injections, which cost about $1,000, are painful and have to be done every six months. Needless to say, Botox injections are substandard care, expensive, and not permanent.

But now there is a permanent cure available! It's called miraDry. The procedure uses microwave energy to heat and destroy the odor and sweat glands of the armpit. Only 85% of patients need one treatment to each underarm; 15% will need a second procedure four to six months later.

A local anesthetic is used, and the treatment lasts about one hour. There is no downtime, and you can go back to work immediately. There will be local pain and swelling for about twenty-four hours. You'll be instructed to ice it for twenty minutes at a time.

I've been doing the miraDry procedure for over a year now and have been amazed at the results for my patients. Check out MiraDry.com for more information. If you are near the Spokane, Washington, area and want the procedure done, send us an email and use the code TGIIL for a 20% discount; and throw away those worthless deodorants and antiperspirants forever.

Chapter 24

DETOXIFICATION

The wise man ought to realize that health is his most valuable possession.

—Hippocrates

Would you like to experience

- more energy,
- better sleep,
- less joint and muscle pain,
- more weight loss,
- improved concentration and memory, and
- clearer skin?

Then it's time to detoxify!

Toxins are everywhere in our life—in the air we breathe, the food we eat, and the water we drink. We are exposed to 2.5 billion pounds of toxic chemicals each and every year. Our lungs, liver, kidneys, skin, and intestinal tract are responsible for detoxification; but our bodies can accumulate more toxins than we can get rid of. These toxins start to build up and are associated with an increased incidence of chronic disease.

And it starts early! Even in utero, we are building up toxins that are delivered through the umbilical cord, as it delivers a steady stream of pollutants, chemicals, and pesticides to the developing baby. An average American baby is born with 287 toxins, but these are only the ones we can measure. Who knows how many more there are that we don't measure. These include pesticides, petrochemicals, the Teflon chemical PFOA (a known human carcinogen), waste from burning coal, and gasoline, mercury, and chemicals used as flame retardants.

Because it starts so early, before we even take our first breath of life, imagine how much has accumulated over the years of your life. We are living in a sea of toxins, and they are making us fat, fatigued, and foggy as they are destroying our bodies and brains. It's therefore important we do everything we can to keep our bodies clean and detoxified as much as possible.

However, conventional medicine will not acknowledge toxicity as a possible cause of disease, yet in reality, they see it in their practice every day. There's the patient that is frustrated that they can't lose weight and wonders why they're fatigued all the time or why the insomnia that does not respond to treatment. All are commonly seen in a physician's practice and can be due to exposures to toxins.

How do you know if you have a buildup of toxins that can cause symptoms and disease?

Signs that you might have toxic buildup include the following:

- Constipation. You should have a bowel movement one to three times a day to remove toxins from the intestinal tract.
- Fatigue. Constant tiredness is often an indication of toxic burdens.

- Abdominal bloating and gas and/or if you've had your gallbladder removed.
- Chronic bad breath.
- Acne or chronic eczema.
- Foggy thinking and slow reactions.
- Fluid retention.
- Sugar cravings.
- Constant sinus congestion.
- Headaches.
- Difficulty losing weight.
- Eczema, acne, and other rashes.
- Moodiness or irritability.

If you have dental fillings, or amalgams, you have mercury in your teeth, and every time you eat, you release some mercury with every chew. Other sources of mercury include seafood and thimerosal-containing vaccines, such as the flu vaccine.

Other heavy metals can also build up, such as lead, tin, nickel, and cadmium. The toxicity of heavy metals produces a wide range of adverse biological effects, especially to the brain. They are known to contribute to tremor, irritability, depression, anxiety, memory loss, and neuropathy. Heavy metals also target other organs and tissues—your liver, digestive tract, kidneys, bone marrow, heart, pancreas, and thyroid.

Genetically, some of us are better at detoxifying than others. A clue to know if you may be someone that has trouble with detoxification is to look at your toes. If the second toe is longer, then you have a defect in MTHFR, or methylation, and as discussed in chapter, you will not be able to clear toxins as readily as another. You'll also tend to be low in B vitamins. This is a common condition, as 40% of the population has this genetic defect. The way to combat this is to take methylated B vitamins, such as methylfolate and methylcobalamin and TMG or trimethylglycine. This will give you back some of the methyl groups you're lacking.

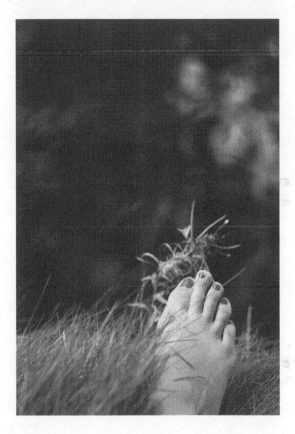

Because toxins also build up and store in fat cells, whenever you lose weight, the toxins are released and can make you sick. These toxins can make it more difficult to lose weight because the body will try to inhibit further fat reduction to reduce toxicity. You don't want this to happen. Of course, you want to eliminate the chemicals and toxins as much as possible.

One way the body does this is a process called glucuronidation. This is where toxins that are released from cells are made water soluble to be eliminated by the kidneys. Without this process, toxins that are fat soluble, which are many, remain in body fat. When you lose weight, the toxins that are released will either be eliminated, or if they remain, your body will want to store them back inside a fat cell and may even create more fat cells to do it! This can be one of the causes of rebound weight gain.

A detoxification protocol can help with weight loss, among other things. It can also significantly improve insulin sensitivity and metabolic syndrome, decreasing your risk of diabetes. There are things we can do every day to help reduce our toxic burden that are not difficult to do. Besides, of course, trying to clean up the diet as we've talked about already and eating organic as much as possible, there are other simple ways to reduce toxins.

For the GI (gastrointestinal) tract, make sure you're eating plenty of fiber and having at least one bowel movement a day. Avoid starchy and high-carb foods. If you tend toward constipation, increase the consumption of raw vegetables and fruit, including prunes, blueberries, tomatoes, and carrots. Use a fiber such as Metamucil or Citrucel daily.

The best foods for detoxification are cruciferous vegetables. This includes broccoli, cauliflower, kale, radish, brussels sprout, cabbage, and garlic. Cilantro is also an excellent spice/food to help us detoxify. Use this liberally.

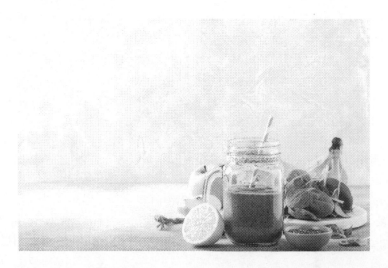

For the kidneys, be sure you're drinking enough water, though this can be difficult on the road since you don't want frequent bathroom breaks. Alkalinize your urine by squeezing lemon in the water and using lemon essential oil. Put two to three drops in a liter of water or in sixteen ounces of water, and drink throughout the day. If your urine is dark, that means you're not drinking enough water and that it's too concentrated. You want it more dilute than that—a light yellow color.

Next is the skin. Sweating is, by far, the best way to detox through the skin. With your workouts, it's good to work hard enough to break out into a sweat. Another great way for detoxification is with an infrared sauna. An infrared sauna will heat your tissues several inches deep, which will improve oxygenation and circulation and help mobilize more toxins for excretion. Of course, you can't very well carry a sauna around the truck, so look for one that you can use when you're home for a few days. Even if you're able to use one once a month, it will be helpful.

The lungs are often forgotten as an organ for detoxification, but they are extremely important in this role. They never stop working day or night (thank goodness!) to give you oxygen and eliminate carbon dioxide with every breath.

In your profession, you'll breathe in fumes from the diesel, fumes from exhaust pipes that surround you from other trucks, harmful germs, and air pollution. And if you smoke, the amount of pollutants with every breath of a cigarette is astronomical.

A simple way for clearing the lungs is to lie down at night and to take deep breaths. Put your hands on your rib cage, and feel the breath expanding your ribs. Count to five as you inhale deeply through your nose. Hold your breath for two seconds, then exhale slowly to the count of five. Repeat ten times, twice a day.

Oregano oil is helpful for clearing the lungs. I use oregano essential oil in a diffuser, but in the cab of your truck, you can simply put one to two drops, and you'll breathe in the scent. Use oregano liberally in cooking as well.

Other spices that are good for lung detox are ginger and peppermint. Peppermint tea is delicious. You can brew it and drink it hot or cold.

Eat foods that are high in vitamin C, such as citrus fruit, kiwi, broccoli, pomegranate, and berries. Eat foods that have a lot of antioxidants, such as garlic, onion, ginger, oregano, and green tea.

And lastly, the liver. The liver is the largest organ in the body, besides the skin, and is often not appreciated, but without it, we cannot survive. Sitting in the right upper quadrant under the rib cage, it has over five hundred vital functions. And it is the most important organ for detoxification.

How do you know if you're liver is toxic?

If you've had your gallbladder taken out, your liver needs help and suffers from bile congestion.

If you're on any medications, *any* of them will stressed your liver. Most meds are metabolized through the liver, and the more meds you're on, the more work it does.

If you have more than just love handles in the abdomen and are carrying a spare tire, you likely have fatty liver. An indication of fatty liver is an elevated liver function test known as ALT. If your ALT is more than 20, you have a stressed liver. Fatty infiltration of the liver is the most common liver disease we see now and can cause liver failure, so it is to be taken seriously. Work on losing the spare tire, and take supplements such as milk thistle that are protective for this organ.

If you drink alcohol, the liver is stressed as it is the organ that works to detoxify any alcohol. A man should not drink more than one alcoholic drink a day; and a woman, a half glass of wine, as any more than this will be difficult to metabolize, especially as we age.

Think of the liver as an oil filter of your truck. The filter can become dirty and congested with old dirty oil, and if not changed regularly, the engine will not run efficiently and will eventually break down. The same thing happens to your liver. It can become congested and toxic. This will add abdominal fat, make you lethargic, make digestion more difficult, and cause abdominal bloating.

So what do we do as a daily routine to detoxify?

1. Drink lemon water daily, and use lemon essential oil.
2. Do deep breathing exercises twice a day.
3. Reduce carbs in the diet to reduce abdominal fat.
4. Eat organic as much as possible, and eat plenty of raw vegetables and fruit.
5. Use EMF protection as discussed in chapter.
6. Sweat a lot in your workout, at least five days a week.
7. Use tourmaline, worn against the skin, as a simple and natural way to detoxify.
8. Quit smoking by all means.

In addition, I recommend a complete detox once every six months. There are different ways to do this, but I like to keep things simple. There's a protocol made by Xymogen that I recommend doing every six months. However, a word of caution. If you consider yourself to be a sensitive or delicate person who reacts to many things, you might have to take things more slowly. This sensitivity could be due to a high exposure to toxins or to a genetically reduced ability to detoxify. Remember the second toe being longer than the first, or big, toe? If you have that, then you have the genetic defect in methylation and can't clear toxins easily. So if you're this person (the sensitive one), the rule "Start low, go slow" is the best way to detox.

The detoxification protocol involves the use of four products.

ProbioMax Daily DF. This is a dairy- and gluten-free probiotic with thirty billion per capsule. This provides four strains of beneficial bacteria that have proven health benefits and help repair the intestinal health.

OptiCleanse GHI. This is a vegetarian amino acid blend with phytonutrients, extra B vitamins, and the following:

- Green tea catechins (support antioxidant activity and detoxification)
- Choline (helps with fat metabolism)
- Ellagic acid from pomegranate extract (increases glutathione, binds directly to toxins, and protects DNA and liver cells)
- Fiber (supports healthy intestinal flora)
- Glutamine (helps with healthy intestinal cell proliferation and gut-barrier integrity)
- Antioxidants such as bioflavonoids, quercetin, rutin, and curcumin (counter free radicals and support healthy cell metabolism)

ColonX. This helps support gastrointestinal regularity and regular bowel movements. It's a mixture of magnesium citrate to help you move things along, cape aloe to add bulk to stool, and a blend of astringent fruits that help digestion and elimination. Warning: if you have bowel movements every day without difficulty, you may not need this product!

Drainage. This combines homeopathic remedies that helps with liver, kidney, and colon functions.

So here's how to do the every six-month detox protocol.

Two days before starting the diet and shakes, do the following:

1. Swallow two capsules of ColonX with water at bedtime. If constipation isn't really an issue, take one capsule of ColonX instead of two.

2. Each morning and evening, place six drops of Drainage on your tongue for ten minutes before or thirty minutes after eating or brushing your teeth.

On days 3–5, continue to take one to two capsules of ColonX at bedtime and continue the six drops of Drainage twice a day. Then add one capsule of ProbioMax with water either at bedtime or in the morning.

Start your OptiCleanse GHI shakes twice a day—for breakfast and dinner.

A large part of your cleanse involves dietary changes. Eliminate certain foods from your diet that may be commonly seen as allergens or sensitivities or that may interfere with your body's natural detoxification processes. You may look at the list and start thinking of the foods you can't have, but don't! There are many delicious foods you *can* have. Cleansing your body of toxins isn't about deprivation or starving yourself; it's about making small improvements in your diet to improve your health. We want to focus on good, whole foods, such as fresh or frozen fruits and vegetables and lean sources of protein, while eliminating those foods that only contribute to inflammation, pain, and fatigue.

As much as you're able, buy foods that are organic, locally grown, and non-GMO. Your meat should be grass-fed, free-range protein sources, and fish should be wild fish from cold, deep waters, never farmed fish. It is more expensive to eat organic, and if your budget or circumstances don't allow you to always eat organic foods, be aware that some foods have more pesticides than others. There's a list called the Dirty 12, meaning the foods that concentrate the most pesticides, and the Clean 15, the foods that have the least. If you can, only buy organic foods if they are part of the Dirty 12. Look at the image below.

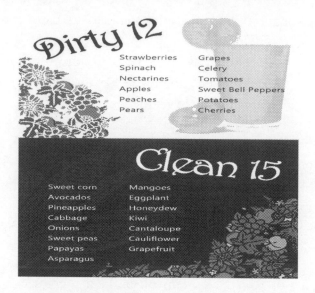

Dirty 12

Strawberries	Grapes
Spinach	Celery
Nectarines	Tomatoes
Apples	Sweet Bell Peppers
Peaches	Potatoes
Pears	Cherries

Clean 15

Sweet corn	Mangoes
Avocados	Eggplant
Pineapples	Honeydew
Cabbage	Kiwi
Onions	Cantaloupe
Sweet peas	Cauliflower
Papayas	Grapefruit
Asparagus	

What do you eat during these five days? Good protein, plenty of vegetables, fresh fruits, nuts, and good oils. See the table below.

Table of foods to remove/ foods to eat:

Foods to Avoid	Foods to Eat
• Alcohol	• Dairy alternatives
• Beef	• Fish
• Chocolate	• Fruits (only those
• Coffee, soft drinks, tea	specifically listed)
• Corn	• Game meats
	• Gluten-free whole grains
	(amaranth, buckwheat,
• Dairy Products	millet, quinoa, rice, teff,
• Eggs	etc.)
• Gluten-containing grains	• Healthy oils
(all varieties of barley,	• Legumes (except soy, peanuts)
rye, spelt, wheat)	• Nuts (except peanuts)
• Peanuts	
• Pork	• Poultry
• Processed meats	• Seeds
• Shellfish	• Vegetables
• Soy and soy products	
Sugar (white sugar,	
high-fructose corn	
syrup, brown sugar,	
sucrose, etc.)	

If you're trying to lose weight, drink the shakes twice a day and only eat one meal a day, preferably lunch. If weight loss is not a goal or is not as important, you can take the shakes twice a day plus eat some of the foods listed on the right above, avoiding the foods on the left.

During this time, water is essential for hydration and a successful cleanse. A good rule of thumb is to take your weight, divide it in half, and consume that number in ounces of water per day. So a two hundred-pound person should drink one hundred ounces of water daily.

Exercise is also an important part of a healthy cleanse. But in this case, keep your exercise routine mild, such as brisk walking or light cardio, avoiding anything strenuous.

The other important component of your detoxification is rest. At night while we sleep, it's essential to get seven to eight hours a night to allow our body to go into repair mode. And getting adequate sleep can help decrease cravings for carbs and sugary foods. Have you noticed how much hungrier you are when you don't get enough sleep?

I recommend this detox protocol every six months. In between, drink one OptiCleanse GHI a day for regular detoxification and added protein. They come in several flavors: vanilla, chai, chocolate mint, and creamy chocolate. Buy a small blender for the truck, something like the magic bullet or other small blender. Here are some delicious formulas:

Berry Shake

10 oz. of cold water
1–2 oz. of crushed ice
1 scoop of vanilla OptiCleanse GHI
5 frozen blackberries and 5 blueberries
7 pecans

Blend and enjoy!

Cherry Vanilla Shake

2 scoops of vanilla OptiCleanse GHI
8 frozen cherries
1 cup of water
34 ice cubes

Blend and enjoy!

Pumpkin Pie Spice Shake

1½ cups of ice and water (or cold decaf coffee)
1 scoop of vanilla OptiCleanse GHI
1/8 tsp. of pumpkin pie spice

Blend and enjoy!

Chai Tea Shake

2 scoops of vanilla OptiCleanse GHI
½ cup of liquid chai tea
½ cup of water
5–6 ice cubes

Blend and enjoy!

Chapter 25

TOURMALINE GEMSTONE

Until I got into the antiaging world of medicine, I had never heard of tourmaline. But now I wear it every day, 24-7. What is it?

Tourmaline is a type of gemstone that is similar to granite. It comes in many different colors and actually changes colors when exposed to light. The word *tourmaline* means "stone mixed with vibrant colors." From blue to maroon to yellow or black, some say that there are no two tourmaline gemstones with the exact same color, and for this reason, it has held a mystical magic power to protect anyone who wears it.

But the real reason it seems to be "magic" is that it has an incredible ability to aid in detoxification. It is only one of a few minerals that have this ability, and it does so by emitting negative ions and far-infrared rays. In other words, it has the ability to become its own source of electric charge.

This charge and infrared rays penetrate the skin and mind and, indeed, can penetrate all layers of the human body, including organs, tissues, muscles, and bones. The far-infrared rays that the gem emits create the same resonance in the body as is found in water. Since the body is composed of three-fourths water, this resonance creates increased vitality, increased energy, and increased metabolism!

Tourmaline has been shown to increase mental alertness, strengthen the immune system, calm the nerves, relieve stress, and help the body detoxify. It is a powerful agent for reducing toxin-related ailments. It helps detoxify even at the deepest tissue level.

By improving circulation, it promotes oxygenation and regeneration of the blood and body.

Another benefit of tourmaline is that it can help significantly with depression. As an example of this, have you ever walked outside after a thunderstorm? Remember the tingly sensation you get and the lift in your mood you experience? That's because of all the negative ions created during a storm, which increase the oxygen flow to the brain, increasing mental awareness and helping improve our moods and outlook on life.

And if this weren't good enough, the gemstone has also been reported to boost the sexual energy of men because of the improvement in circulation. It increases the vitality and vigor in both men and women.

So to sum it up, the benefits of tourmaline are that it

- provides detoxification for the liver, kidneys, and skin;
- improves circulation;
- enhances immunity;
- clears the skin;
- helps with fat loss and metabolism;
- improves sleep;
- increases energy;
- improves mood and reduces depression;
- aids in elimination of heavy metals and other toxins;
- reduces water retention; and
- accelerates recovery time from injuries to muscles, tendons, and bones.

With all these benefits, tourmaline should be included in your daily detoxification protocol. It is so easy to use and produces the best effects when your body is in close proximity or against the skin. I wear a bracelet that has the tourmaline against the skin. It doesn't rust or tarnish, even with water, and it does not lose its power with time.

There are many companies advertising tourmaline, but like anything, you have to be careful of quality. The only company I trust with the quality needed for tourmaline bracelets is Nano-Ions.com. There are some made for both men and women. Put in code to get a special reduced price of $149. Unlike a vitamin that you have to buy each month, this is a one-time purchase, and it lasts forever, continuing its health benefits as long as it's worn.

Chapter 26

ANTIAGING MEDICINE

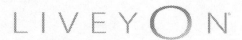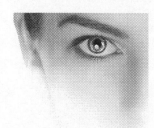

Make today so awesome that yesterday gets jealous!

I practiced traditional, Western medicine for twenty years and noticed a pattern. There was a large group of patients for which I had no answers and could offer no help. These were the patients with chronic fatigue, inability to lose weight, chronic pain and stiffness, muscle wasting, autoimmune disease, and depression. Drugs did not help, and they often made things worse. Or one drug caused side effects that required two more drugs to be prescribed. And then they caused side effects, and more drugs were prescribed, which caused . . . You see the problem.

So I started looking for more, something else that could help my patients. I found a new specialty called antiaging and regenerative medicine, went back to school, and obtained a second board certification in this field.

What is integrative or regenerative medicine? This is a branch of medicine that is aimed at getting to the root cause of the disease or symptoms, slowing down the rate of aging, and improving the quality of life as we get older. It's about restoring you to your optimal health—restoring vitality, improving energy, and regaining the spark of life that so often fades as we age.

If you are tired all the time, you are not aging well, and it is a sign that something, internally, has gone awry.

If you have belly fat that seems impossible to get rid of, you are not aging well. Your liver is stressed and is unable to clear toxins efficiently, causing them to be stored in fat instead.

If you have frequent heartburn, gas, and/or bloating, you are not aging well, with an unhealthy gut creating an unhealthy body.

If you are on three or more medications, you are not aging well, with the meds often having systemic side effects that can affect every organ in the body.

If you can't get to sleep or wake up frequently during the night, you are not aging well, and this will act as a chronic stressor to your body, making it deteriorate more quickly.

If your joints are stiff and sore and it hurts to walk, sit, or stand, you are not aging well; and that is a sign that things are wearing out.

If your ambition and motivation are low and you would rather sit in front of a TV instead of seizing the day, you are not aging well, and the vitality and spark of life are being dimmed.

And if you'd like to turn this around, find a doctor that is trained in integrative and functional medicine. She or he can start the general assessment of your health and start you on the path to health.

Start making the dietary changes needed as discussed in previous chapters, and begin taking high-quality vitamins to pour in the nutrition your body—your machine—requires.

Consider seeing an excellent chiropractor in your area to check for any spinal misalignments that can impede your health.

Make exercise a regular part of your life, even if you've never exercised before. Start with walking a few laps around your truck. Work up to using some basic exercise equipment, the bands, stair stepper, vibration plate—whatever you have in your possession. Make muscles that haven't worked in a long time work. Without exercise that's consistently performed day after day, week after week, year after year, you will age much more quickly.

It's amazing how the simple things, the ones your mama probably told you to do, are the ones that keep us the healthiest. Eat right, exercise, keep your weight down, and take your vitamins.

But if you want to be even more aggressive about turning back the hand of time, consider stem cell therapy, which we'll discuss in the next chapter.

Chapter 27

STEM CELLS

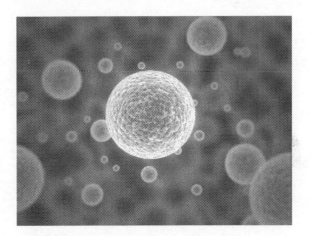

What has the potential to change the way we practice medicine in the next ten years? What has the potential to actually grow new cells, repair cartilage, bones, and organs, including heart, kidneys, lungs, and neurological tissues? Stem cells.

What, exactly, are stem cells? You might have heard something about them by now. Basically, a stem cell has the potential to become any cell. It's like having a blank slate that can be carved into whatever statue you need. Maybe it's that torn cartilage in your knee, and the orthopedic surgeon has said you'll need a knee replacement. Or it's emphysema, lung tissue damaged by years of smoking, that's now being repaired and lung capacity increasing. Or it's congestive heart failure, dying heart cells that are no longer an effective pump, that's now being repaired with new heart cells to replace the damaged areas.

And even more profound is a patient with a spinal cord injury, paralyzed and in a wheelchair, now able to walk and have control over bowels and bladder.

These sound like miracles, don't they? They may well be, and they represent the power of stem cells.

We all believe that stem cells are new, but in reality, they've been used since 1956, when the world's first bone marrow transplant was performed between identical twins, where one had leukemia.

Stem cells can be from three different sources:

1. *Embryonic stem cell*s. These are derived from the tissue of embryos, often fetal tissue that are often from abortions. There are obvious ethical and moral dilemmas and legal repercussions with this. These may be used in other countries, but not ours. Embryonic stem cells have the potential to form tumors, as the cells continue to try to form a baby and instead form masses of tissue. I never recommend this type of stem cell for moral, ethical, legal, and safety reasons.

2. *Autologous stem cells*. These are derived from your own tissue. These are most often obtained from either fat cells or bone marrow. While these may work, the problem with them is that they are as old as you are and are therefore not as potent. Also, since stem cells are attracted to areas of inflammation, they may be directed to the areas where the fat was extracted or where the bone marrow needle was inserted instead of the areas that you want and truly need them. The

procedure is invasive, painful, and is not one I generally recommend.

3. *Umbilical stem cells.* These are derived from the umbilical cords from healthy babies. The procedure is as follows: when a cesarean section is planned, the mother is asked if she wants to bank her baby's umbilical cord blood. This is an expensive process, and it is usually declined. They are then asked if they will donate the umbilical cord, and if they agree, the technician from the lab will be there at the time of the cesarean section and obtain the cord within one hour. The blood is then extracted and screened for many diseases, and stem cells are derived from them.

I recommend umbilical cord stem cells as they are the most potent, being zero days old, and the procedure is noninvasive, safe, and easy to perform. There are also no side effects such as tumor growth associated with embryonic stem cells and no moral or ethical dilemmas.

An important thing to realize about umbilical cord cells is that they are a type of immature cell that the immune system doesn't recognize as foreign, so they will not trigger rejection. They are also more energetic than other types of stem cells and, therefore, have a better chance of persisting, reducing inflammation, and being more effective.

I use stem cells in my antiaging and regenerative medicine practice as an IV infusion, and I inject it directly in joints when needed. I have seen profound results with the umbilical cord stem cells used in my practice. Some examples include the following:

My own husband, who had a tear of his medial meniscus of his knee, was told by orthopedics that he'd eventually need surgery. After an injection over this area, he completely healed the tear and was able to walk without pain. In addition, the cartilage space increased, with the hope of avoiding a knee replacement in his future.

A fifty-eight-year-old female with a chronic lung condition that was progressive, with nothing more that could be offered by Western medicine is now with a 35% higher lung capacity and a reduction in wheezing after two IV infusions.

Osteoarthritis of the thumb, causing pain with every movement, even grasping or twisting, was completely resolved after one IV infusion.

There was a sixty-year-old man with congestive heart failure resulting from a heart attack, with his heart functioning at 25% capacity. He was short of breath with every step and was on a number of drugs from cardiology. After one IV infusion, his ejection fraction increased from 20% to 45%, and he felt like his life was back. A normal ejection fraction is between 50% and 70%. A repeat stem cell infusion three months later increased his ejection fraction to 55%. He plans on having a yearly infusion for the indeterminate future.

There are many other patients with orthopedic conditions, diabetes, autoimmune diseases, respiratory disorders, and frailty who have been helped with umbilical cord stem cell treatments. To see if you are a candidate for stem cells, call our office at 509-924-6199. An evaluation can be done in person or (we know you're busy driving across the country) can also be done over the phone. The infusion itself takes about a half hour, and you'll be on your way again. At this time, it is not covered by insurance, but it costs much less than the price of a joint replacement or other chronic conditions.

Chapter 28

ENERGY MEDICINE

Don't call it a dream. Call it a plan.

Conventional or Western medicine tends to focus on using chemicals that affect organs, tissues, and cells, such as drugs that lower blood pressure, increase serotonin, and lower stomach acid. These chemicals are inherently foreign to our bodies and often cause side effects that require more medications to treat.

Energy medicine, on the other hand, looks at and measures the effects of energy fields and how they affect the growth and repair processes on cells, tissues, and organs. Things that include energy medicine include acupuncture, tai chi, qigong, yoga, reflexology, and kinesiology.

Western medicine and our society in general tend to ignore the effects of our emotional state and the role that it plays in nearly every physical disease. Heart disease, cancer, irritable bowel, arthritis, kidney disease, and more all can result from or be made worse by any blocked emotions or mental illness.

Even the CDC (Centers for Disease Control) has reported that 85% of all diseases have an emotional element. And a twenty-year study conducted by the University of London found that unmanaged stress is a *more serious* risk factor for both heart disease and cancer than either cigarette smoking or frequent consumption of high-cholesterol foods.

Our emotions can also change our genetic expression, turning genes on or off. So for example, you've inherited a gene that will increase your risk of, say, colon cancer, that gene might remain unexpressed or turned off for your entire life; and you never actually get colon cancer. But if a powerful, emotional event occurs that is not dealt with, leading to blocked emotions, this can change the gene expression, turn the gene on, and therefore, colon cancer will now occur.

Blocked emotions can affect energy fields of the body, such as the meridian lines that acupuncture works on. Depending on which energy fields are blocked, this can lead to symptoms and a multitude of diseases. Every trapped emotion, no matter what age they occurred or how big or small, can impact you in some way. And the emotions can even be inherited up to seven generations back. Let's say you have had a wonderful childhood, two parents that loved you, good neighborhoods and schools, and nothing more than the usual childhood illnesses and bumps and scrapes. But for some reason, you simply cannot pinpoint that you have this underlying anxiety that is hampering your life—a feeling of panic at times, something that has you grinding your teeth, irritable bowel, fatigue, and insomnia. But why?

Consider that it may be the result of how your great-great-great-great-grandfather endured a hardship, perhaps famine or war or abuse, and this left such an impact that it created something called a blocked emotion. This blocked emotion disrupted different energy fields and was passed down through generations, just like DNA.

If you are interested in learning more about this, I highly encourage you to read the book called *The Emotion Code* by Dr. Bradley Nelson.

It is profound, and I believe Dr. Nelson was given this gift by God to benefit mankind. With this book, you will learn how to identify your own blocked emotions and release them yourself and be able to perform this for your family.

Another technique that is used in energy medicine is called emotional freedom technique or EFT. This one is also great, and I want each one of you to learn it, as it's so easy but yet powerful in improving our emotional health. Remember, no matter how physically healthy you are—eating right and exercising, keeping your weight down— you will not achieve optimal health if you continue to have blocked emotional barriers impeding the natural healing potential of the body.

EFT is an acupressure technique based on the energy meridians used in acupuncture for thousands of years, but without using needles. Instead, you use your fingertips and a simple tapping method to put kinetic energy back into the meridians that help you clear negative emotions while replacing them with positive affirmations. This helps to clear the emotional blocks from your body's bioenergetic system.

EFT works. It has a high rate of success, and its use has spread throughout the world. The technique is easy to do and only takes a few minutes to learn and perform. The best free resource is on YouTube. Just search for EFT or emotional freedom technique. You'll be able to watch and have it down in no time at all.

EFT is done by tapping with your fingertips of the index and middle fingers with one hand. It doesn't matter which hand, either one works. You can also use both hands and all your fingers. This will allow you to access more acupuncture points. If you do use both hands, alternate the tapping with both hands simultaneously. You will tap at specific points that represent acupressure points of the body. At each point, you'll tap between five to eight times or about the length of time it takes to complete one full breath.

You'll start at the head and work your way down to the underarm area. Remove glasses, watches, and bracelets prior to starting, as they can interfere with electromagnetic fields.

The tapping points are shown below.

(See pics.)

1. Top of the head.
2. Edge of inner eyebrows.
3. Side of the eye (temple area).
4. Under the eye (on the bone about one inch below the pupil).
5. Between the nose and upper lip.
6. Chin.
7. Collarbone. Find the site where your collarbone meets your sternum or breastbone. Just under this area is a very powerful acupuncture area known as *K*. Move down one inch from this spot.
8. Four inches below the armpit.
9. Inside of both wrists.

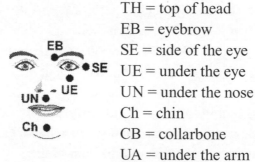

TH = top of head
EB = eyebrow
SE = side of the eye
UE = under the eye
UN = under the nose
Ch = chin
CB = collarbone
UA = under the arm
WR = wrists

Now for the wording part. First, identify the problem you want focus on. Let's take anxiety as an example. Next, you'll want to make a statement to acknowledge the problem, then follow it with an unconditional affirmation of yourself. For example,

Even though I _____, I deeply and completely accept myself.

So in this instance, it would be "Even though I feel this anxiety, I deeply and completely accept myself" or "Even though I feel panic when thinking about ___, I deeply and completely accept myself." Repeat the statement three times while simultaneously tapping each point.

It may seem silly at first, and you'll probably want to do this in private to keep others from thinking you've gone off the deep end. But it can truly be effective as a universal healing tool for both physical and emotional issues.

Next is EMF (electromagnetic fields). We've all heard about the dangerous effects of EMF—that they can cause cancer, neurological diseases, and other health problems. The EPA has labeled magnetic fields a class-3 carcinogen. But the truth is, of course, much more complicated than that.

We are highly tuned and highly sensitive bioelectrical animals. Every cell has its own electromagnetic field, and our body is regulated by electrical currents.

We are all exposed to EMF, even if you live in a jungle with no electronics. The very planet we live on exposes us to EMF, and each one of us makes a small amount of EMF. Every living and nonliving thing emits its own electromagnetic fields. A small amount of EMF is not bad for us, and in fact, it may be good for us. As with everything, it's the *overexposure* of EMF that is hazardous. Too much of anything is not good for us.

The EMF we are bombarded with on a daily basis comes from

1. cell phones;
2. computers;
3. Wi-Fi;
4. light bulbs;
5. the sun;
6. appliances (microwaves, blenders, hair dryers, TVs);
7. wireless devices (cordless phones, baby monitors, security cameras);
8. electric clock radios;
9. the power meter outside your house;
10. cell towers; and
11. wireless routers.

Cordless phones are a major source of EMF and should never be by your sleeping area. You want the cordless phone at least three rooms away from where you are sleeping. The base of the phone transmits constantly, whether it is being used or not. When speaking in either a cordless phone or a cell phone, it is best to use them on speaker mode or with a headset. Never carry a cell phone in your pocket or next to your skin.

Symptoms of overexposure to EMF are fatigue, headaches, mental dullness (foggy brain), insomnia, reduced sperm count and motility, heart palpitations, dizziness, tingling, depression of the immune system causing susceptibility to colds and flu, anxiety, and other behavioral problems.

If you've had a joint replacement, the metal, such as titanium, can make you even more sensitive to EMF. The metal acts as a receiver of sorts, attracting the radiation that is constantly bombarding us.

What can you do to protect yourself from EMF? The easiest products that are most effective are energydots. They're about the size of a dime, and I peel off the adhesive backing and apply it to my watch or other jewelry that I wear every day. SmartDOTs can be applied to any electrical device you use every day, such as your cell phone or computer.

For the cab of your truck, use a spaceDOT. The spaceDOT continuously radiates a Phi energy to interact resonantly with your environment to produce a powerful clearing harmonic. The harmonic reenergizes and balances the area and is perfect for the cab of your truck or your home and how far they extend from their source.

You can also purchase an electropollution detector to tell you how strong EMF radiation waves are and how far they radiate beyond the device.

When purchasing a cell phone, know your SAR (specific absorption rate). SAR measures the amount of radiation the phone puts out. The lower the SAR, the better. Anything higher than a 0.5 is too high. The iPhone 7 has the highest, with an SAR of 1.13–1.3. I put a smartDOT on my cell phone for protection.

Try earthing. Never heard of it? Earthing, also known as grounding, is what happens when we go barefoot through the grass or run barefoot on the beach with the sand between our toes. Remember how good that feels? You probably didn't know that you were being protected from EMF radiation by absorbing electrons from the earth. The earth's electrons are conducted to your body, bringing it to the same electrical potential as the earth. Direct contact with the earth grounds your body, which helps us to feel more energized and induces favorable electrophysiological changes that promote optimum health.

There is much evidence to support earthing's improvements in our health, including reducing inflammation, improving heart rate variability and sleep, and enhancing the immune system. It is a great stress reliever.

So weather permitting, try placing your bare feet on the ground, whether it be grass, sand, dirt, or concrete, especially when it is humid or wet. Twenty minutes a day is best. Walking on asphalt or wood does not work, as they are natural insulators.

But when the demands of work do not allow such luxuries, there are other ways. An earthing mat will do the trick. You can purchase these inexpensively to put on your desk to lie on, sit on, or put your bare feet on when you're settled down for the night. Try it, and you might find yourself calmer, more resistant to disease, sleeping better at night, and having more energy during the day.

Section Five

SUPPLEMENTS AND EXERCISE

Chapter 29

SUPPLEMENTS

Choosing to be positive and have a grateful attitude is going to determine how you're going to live your life.

I've discussed in previous chapters the importance of various vitamins and supplements for our health. The older we get, the less nutrients we absorb from our food, and that's even with a perfect diet. Add the fact that our diet is not perfect, especially as a long-haul truck driver, and multiple vitamin deficiencies start adding up, leading to chronic disease. Osteoarthritis of the knees and other joints, diabetes, heart disease, constant tiredness—these are all signs of nutrient deficiencies.

Let's start with the basics. Your vitamins should be medical or pharmaceutical grade and *not* food-grade vitamins. Most vitamins are poorly absorbed, often have contaminants, and many times do not have what their labels say they have. One study of the supplements sold at GNC, Walgreens, and Walmart found that four out of five products didn't contain the ingredient they claimed. So the bottom line is, be picky about your vitamins, and do not waste money on supplements that do not work.

I recommend the following for everyone:

The Basics

Multivitamin. A good multi should have the right kind of nutrients. Vitamin E should always contain mixed tocopherols. Vitamin B6 should be pyridoxal-5'-phosphate, folate should be methyltetrahydrofolic acid, and B12 should be methylcobalamin. Magnesium should *not* be oxide. If you are not a woman having monthly periods, you usually don't need iron.

Fish oil. Unless you live in Alaska and are eating salmon every day, you are deficient in omega-3s. The omega-3s are important for joint health and help to reduce inflammation and lower risks of heart disease, stroke, arthritis, and cancer. They are highly concentrated in the brain and are important for cognitive health, protecting our brain from dementia and Parkinson's. On average, we need between 3,000 and 4,000 mg a day. Since most fish oil capsules have 1,000 mg, that means taking three to four caps a day, which is what I always did until I found one called MonoPure. It's made by Xymogen, and the omega-3s in MonoPure are more highly absorbed than other brands, and one 1,300 mg capsule is equivalent to 3,000 mg of other brands. I take one 1,200 mg in the morning and a smaller 650 mg at night with food. The fish oil is also pure, with all the mercury and other toxins removed. Since our seafood is contaminated with methylmercury and other toxins, a company must spend the money to extract these from their product, and many companies choose not to do so. Be very careful about your fish oil product because you do not want to be ingesting mercury every day!

Vitamin D. No matter where you live, you are most likely low in vitamin D. In all my years of practice, I can remember only a handful of patients that were not low in D, and these were young and very healthy people. We live in Washington state, and everyone here is low in D. But in the south, Florida and Texas for example, most are low in D too. Why is that? We don't know for certain, but it has been hypothesized that the use of sunscreens are causing permanent changes in our skin, with not allowing the absorption of D from the sun. And of course, most of us are working indoors or wearing sunscreen in the summer, which blocks D absorption.

The health benefits of vitamin D are so numerous that if you can afford only one vitamin, this would be it. People with higher D levels have lower age-related changes in their DNA, along with lower inflammation. Optimal levels are between 70 and 90. Normal on lab is listed as 30, but do not accept a level of 30. When D levels are in the 70–90 range, health benefits include lower heart disease risk, less fatigue and joint pain, protection from osteoporosis, less cancer risk, and a stronger immune system. It will slash cancer risks by 60%. I normally take 10,000 IU of D-3 in the winter and 5,000 IU in the summer. Take D with food containing some fat or oil, as it's best absorbed with oil. I take mine with my fish oil in the morning.

Some doctors prescribe a vitamin D as a 50,000 IU capsule to take once a week. I don't recommend this because this form of D is D-2, not D-3. D-2 is not absorbed as readily and must be converted to D-3 to be effective in our body. Take D-3 instead.

To make it easy, I've combined a multivitamin and mineral supplement with D-3 5,000 and a 1,300 mg of MonoPure capsule in one packet. It's so easy to take—one packet daily. Great for travel, and it is pharmaceutical grade.

Specialty Supplements

Adrenal Manager. This is an exceptional product for adrenal fatigue. If you have constant fatigue, wake up tired, crave sugar and/or salt, then you may well have adrenal fatigue, meaning the cortisol levels are low. The only accurate way to diagnose this is with a saliva test, measuring cortisol levels four times throughout the day. Try Adrenal Manager; take two capsules daily. Don't take past 3:00 pm, or it can cause insomnia.

B Activ. This is a B complex that has the entire spectrum of B vitamins with the activated forms of B2, B6, folate, and B12. If you have a high homocysteine level, you need extra B vitamins; take one twice daily. If you notice more energy with this B vitamin, that means you are low in the Bs, so continue to take one to two per day.

ATP Ignite. This is a great energy drink. Each stick contains B vitamins, electrolytes, minerals, amino acids, herbs, and antioxidants to fuel your body's energy production. It also contains caffeine that is slowly absorbed over eight hours. Use it for when you need a little extra energy or for your workouts.

ALAmax Protect. This contains berberine and ALA to reduce insulin resistance, lower blood sugar and A1C, and help with glucose metabolism. Berberine also helps to lower inflammation and triglycerides. This is a great supplement for anyone with diabetes or prediabetes.

Calcium D-glucarate. This helps the liver detoxify and helps with estrogen metabolism. If you are a man with high estrogen, this can help to detoxify and break this down while also reducing fat soluble toxins. For any weight-loss regimen, I recommend Calcium D-glucarate twice a day for the first three months to help with weight loss and help clear toxins from the liver.

Candicidal. This helps with digestion and eliminates yeast from our intestinal tract. If you've had multiple antibiotics and/or irritable bowel syndrome, then you have yeast. The yeast or candida will make it harder to lose weight and will make you more tired as it will absorb your B vitamins. Take two caps a day.

ColonX. If you have constipation, this supplement works great. It promotes normal GI transit time and supports all phases of digestion and elimination. Take one to two caps at bedtime.

CoQmax. This is CoQ10 at either 100 mg or 200 mg. Take 200 mg if you are on a statin and 100 mg if you are over fifty or have any heart disease. CoQ10 is needed for energy production and is critical for the heart and brain. A side effect of too little CoQ10 is fatigue, cognitive impairment, muscle cramping, and premature aging.

Cortisolv. Are you a very stressed-out person? Feel like you can't relax at night to sleep? Then this is the supplement for you. Take one cap twice a day or two at night.

DIMension 3. This is a critical supplement for estrogen metabolism. Ladies, if you take bioidentical hormones, take DIM to help reduce your levels of estrone, the unhealthy estrogen. DIM may reduce your levels of breast cancer and can help reduce prostate cancer in men.

Femquil. This is the best hormone supplement for women on the market. It helps with estrogen detoxification, reduces PMS, and helps ease symptoms of menopause. It also has great antioxidants that help reduce risk of breast cancer. Take two capsules twice a day for the first three months, and if symptoms have diminished or resolved, try reducing to one twice a day.

GI Protect. This is an excellent supplement for irritable bowel syndrome, leaky gut, and multiple food allergies or sensitivities. It helps heal the lining of the GI tract and supports the immune system. Take one scoop twice daily.

Immune Essentials. Do you have frequent colds and flus? If so, this is the supplement for you. It has powerful beta-glucan, which keeps the immune system healthy and strong. Add vitamin C and olive leaf extract, and you've got a powerful formula. Take one a day as prevention or three a day on an empty stomach for a cold or flu.

Iron Glycinate. Take only if you've been diagnosed with iron deficiency—often found in women who have heavy periods. This form of iron is highly absorbed, much better than the more common iron sulfate, and doesn't cause as much constipation with less food interactions.

I-Sight. This is eye support for prevention of macular degeneration or cataracts. Our eyes age and deteriorate just like other organs, and this product can help slow that aging process.

L-lysine. Take daily for prevention of cold sores. Usually one to two a day will do.

Liver Protect. Have you been told you have fatty liver? Do you take daily Tylenol? Drink alcohol more than three days a week? If so, you need Liver Protect. This will help your liver detoxify and allow it to function more efficiently, helping to clear out the huge amount of toxins we're exposed to daily. Take one to two caps a day.

MedCaps Menopause. Ladies, are you having hot flashes that won't let up? I know from personal experience that it can completely disrupt your life or keep you up at night. If you're going through menopause, bioidentical hormones can help, but if you're not on hormones or can't take them, try this product. It has ten ingredients, all that aim to reduce hot flashes and night sweats.

Melatonin. A hormone and an antioxidant, melatonin is the number 1 product for sleep. If you have insomnia, try this. One to two hours before bed is best. If you're over age fifty, you likely need it, as your levels decrease with age. Melatonin will reduce your risk of either prostate or breast cancer, and it helps protect the brain from dementia. In Europe, women with breast cancer are using high doses, between 15 and 20 mg a day, to help reduce the aggressiveness of the tumor. The typical dose for insomnia is between 1 and 5 mg/night, 3 mg on average.

MemorAll. Having problems with your memory? This is the product for you. It has twelve ingredients, all that work to increase brain processing speed and improve memory. Take one cap twice a day.

Methylcobalamin. This is a B12 tablet that dissolves quickly, giving extra B12 for energy. If you are on metformin, a common drug that is used for diabetes, you are low in B12 if you're not supplementing with it. Studies have shown that people that take B12 have longer telomeres than those who don't. B12 is found almost exclusively in animal tissues, so if you are a vegetarian, you are low. Dissolve in mouth once daily.

OptiCleanse. This is a great detox shake. Take two scoops daily for two weeks. Mix with ice and some berries, stevia to sweeten, and drink once a day. Do this every six months, optimally, for detox.

OptiMag. This is a magnesium product that doesn't cause diarrhea. Magnesium is the fourth most abundant mineral in the body and is involved in over 1,300 enzyme processes. This includes processes for bone and teeth, the metabolism of carbohydrates, blood glucose, fats and proteins, the formation of cells and tissues, and maintenance of muscle function. If you are having muscle cramps, it is almost always because of low magnesium. Try this first. Other signs of low magnesium are heart palpitations, a heart rate that is too fast, anxiety, and insomnia. Insufficient levels of magnesium will reduce the body's ability to repair damaged DNA. Take two caps one to two times a day.

Ossopan MD. This give comprehensive bone support. Many women after menopause have low bone density and need bone support. However, the calcium has to be an absorbable type. The most common type of calcium that is sold is calcium carbonate, and this form is poorly absorbed and has been implicated in heart disease. Ossopan contains the world's premium sources of bone that is highly absorbed and essential trace elements for bone support. Take two a day with meals twice a day.

PMS Soothe. This works great for PMS symptoms. Take two caps a day and start one week before your period, and you can usually stop two days after the period starts.

ProbioMax Daily DF. This is a probiotic containing thirty billion probiotics per capsule. Remember, a healthy gut is a healthy body, and if you suffer from IBS or have had multiple antibiotics (more than three), you likely need a probiotic.

ProbioMax 350 DF. This probiotic contains the highest amount of probiotics on the market—one packet has 350 billion! When do we need such a large amount? If you have leaky gut or have had *C. difficile* or other intestinal infections, I recommend you take this for two months, along with a supplement called IG 26. The IG 26 kills the bad bacteria while you're pouring in the good bacteria, and it can be very effective.

ProbioMax DF. This contains one hundred billion probiotics. I recommend taking this once a day for thirty days twice a year—when you do your twice-yearly detox. Take before bedtime so you're not putting food on top of it and for better absorption.

Prostate FLO. If you're a male over age fifty and having signs of an enlarged prostate, this is an excellent supplement. What are the signs of an enlarged prostate? Urinary frequency, having to get up at night to urinate, decreased force of the stream, and going with small amounts at a time. Take one to two daily. It may also help to lower the PSA (prostate test in the blood).

RegeneMax. Ladies, do you have hair loss? Thinning hair? This is the formula for you. I have had great success with it. Take one capsule twice a day for three months.

RelaxMax. Do you have difficulty relaxing at night? Turning your mind off? Getting to sleep quickly? RelaxMax has five ingredients that help with relaxation and a deeper sleep, including magnesium, GABA, and L-theanine. Dissolve one scoop with half a cup of water in the evening.

SAMe and TMG. This is a great product for depression. Often, this works so well that you can avoid antidepressants with it. Take one packet daily. If it is going to help your depression, you will notice a difference within thirty days.

SynovX DJD. Do you have joint pain (osteoarthritis)? If you have knee, low back, hip, or other joint pain, especially while getting in and out of the truck, take this daily to help lower inflammation and pain. This will also help slow the progression of the arthritis. Take two caps daily.

T-150. This is for thyroid support. If you have hypothyroidism, if you've been told your thyroid is borderline, or if the size of your thyroid is enlarged, you need nutrients that are specific for that organ. Take one daily.

UritraX. If you have frequent bladder infections, otherwise known as UTI (urinary tract infection), they are usually caused by *E. coli.* This product has D-mannose, which *E. coli* loves. The bacteria will attach to the D-mannose instead of the bladder wall, and when you urinate, you'll flush the *E. coli* out of your system. Take one teaspoon daily for prevention, and take three times a day when you have an infection.

Zinc Glycinate. Zinc is found in every cell of the body and is a powerful antioxidant. Low levels accelerate aging. It is also vital for maintaining hormone levels, and zinc deficiencies can cause infertility, low libido, and in men, erectile dysfunction. Zinc is critical for testosterone production, and a low level is often the cause of low testosterone.

Symptoms of low zinc include increased respiratory illness, sugar and salt cravings, diarrhea, fatigue, slow wound healing, and ringing in the ears.

Women typically need 20 mg a day, whereas men need between 20 and 60 mg a day.

7-keto DHEA. DHEA is an antiaging hormone that begins to decline at age thirty, and all of us over fifty need this hormone. The 7-keto form of DHEA does not convert to testosterone, so it is great for women who have adequate testosterone levels. Regular DHEA will convert to testosterone. The 7-keto DHEA helps support the immune system, maintains muscle mass, and helps with libido and with fat metabolism. Take between 25 and 100 mg a day.

DHEA. For women, if you need testosterone, take between 5 and 10 mg/day. For men, the dose is between 25 and 50 mg a day on average. If you're over fifty, you need DHEA!

There are many other supplements that are effective for different conditions. Just check our website. The supplements will be mailed directly to you.

Chapter 30

Exercise

Don't watch the clock. Do what it does. Keep going.

We are all drilled from an early age on the importance of exercise. It starts in school in our PE class, where they have you doing jumping jacks, running laps, and counting how many push-ups and sit-ups you can do. Most of us learn to hate it.

But the truth of it is, our bodies were made for movement. We evolved from ancestors who spent their time on the move, looking for food and shelter and traveling for miles on end. Then they would sprint, running to catch food or to avoid becoming food.

We have evolved to be regularly active. We are *not* meant to sit for hours on end, yet this is exactly what happens in your profession. It is the cycle of "objects at rest tend to remain at rest." This is Newton's first law of motion and is true for all of us.

To be healthy, you must, I repeat, *must* exercise! There just isn't any way around this. Why? The following is to remind you of all the reasons we exercise:

1. It increases energy by increasing the oxygen utilization of our muscles. Regular exercise increases energy throughout the day.

2. It relieves stress and depression. Our mood is significantly lifted on days we exercise. The natural endorphins are better than any antidepressant, and we feel better about ourselves. Exercise also helps you feel more confident in yourself.

3. It reduces cardiovascular disease, strengthens the heart muscle, reduces blood pressure, improves HDL (good cholesterol), and reduces LDL (bad cholesterol).

4. It lowers risk of diabetes by reducing blood sugar, reducing fat, and increasing muscle mass.

5. You'll sleep better. Regular exercise can help you sleep better and deeper.

6. It enhances your immune system, allowing your body to better fight virus and bacteria.

7. It improves memory. You think more clearly after exercise, and your brain is better able to memorize and focus.

8. It makes bones stronger. Not only do the muscles get stronger but the bones do too. People who exercise regularly have a greater stimulation of bone cell production. The risks of osteoarthritis also go down.

9. It reduces risks of certain cancers by up to 35%. Being overweight increases your risk of many cancers, such as colon, breast, lung, and endometrial cancers.

10. Your posture improves. Our muscles connect to our bones with tendons and ligaments. People who don't exercise regularly risk muscle atrophy, which can lead to weakness and poor posture.

11. It increase your metabolism by maintaining muscle mass. You'll keep your metabolism higher. Muscles burn many more calories than fat does throughout the day, even while you sleep. The more muscle mass you have, the more calories you burn. Also, after exercise, you will burn more calories for

the next twenty-four hours than if you did with no exercise that day.

12. It makes you smarter. Exercise increases brain mass, especially the area of the brain known as the hippocampus, which is critical for short-term memory. The hippocampus shrinks with Alzheimer's and dementia, and you would like to maintain a healthy hippocampal size with age.

So we have plenty of reasons to exercise, and of course, it all boils down to maintaining our health, keeping our weight down, and slowing the aging process.

I hear the excuses already—"You don't know my work schedule," "I put ten to twelve hours a day in the cab of this truck," "I'm too tired," "There's no place to exercise," "The weather's bad," and "I'll start next week."

But this day is a new day, a day of no excuses, and we start our exercise program today!

The plan is to exercise five days a week. If you want to do seven, fine, but we strive for five.

There are two main types of exercise: aerobic or endurance training and strength or resistance training. Both are important. Men tend to like weight training more, and women tend to prefer cardio training. But each of us needs both types to keep our body functioning at peak performance.

Aerobic exercise gets our heart rate up and burns calories. We need to do aerobic exercise for twenty minutes at a minimum of three days a week, but five is better.

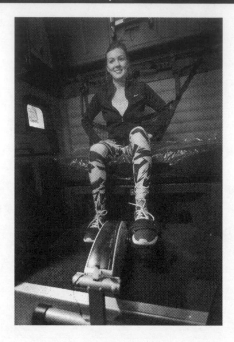

There are small portable exercise equipment that can be purchased and placed in the cab of your truck. These include a stair stepper, DeskCycle, even an elliptical. They can be used in the cab of your truck even on rainy or snowy days.

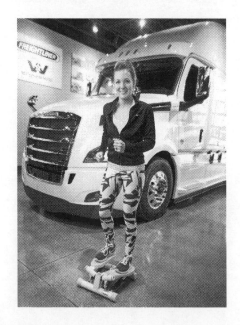

In addition, there are exercises that can be done around your truck that will get your heart rate going. That includes walking around the truck (thirty-two times around a semi is one mile). First thing in the morning, before you start your drive, walk sixteen times around the truck. Get a half mile in before you ever sit down. Park as far away from the truck stop as you can to give you a little extra walking each day.

There are some truck stops, mainly in the South, that have exercise equipment, including bikes and treadmills. If you're lucky enough to be around one of them, stop and get your thirty minutes of exercise that day.

Next, for strength training, you'll want to work on your upper then lower body and also work with core strengthening.

For the upper, the simplest way to build up the arm muscles is push-ups. Do as many as you can at least once a day. If you can't do a regular push-up, do the modified push-up on your knees. (See pic.) Next, do a tricep push-ups. (See pic.)

Dips can be done between the tires, bending at your elbows. If it's raining, use the driver's seat and the passenger's seat to do your dips.

You can also bring some weights with you in the truck. A great brand of portable dumbbells is XMark's adjustable dumbbell. There are numerous exercises that can be done with dumbbells and a good portable set is worth the money.

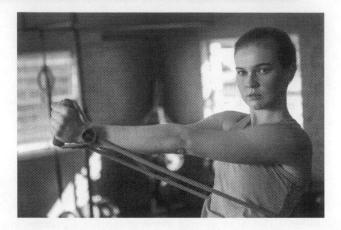

Another alternative is to get a set of resistance bands. There are so many exercises that can be done with a $20 set of bands for the arms, legs, abs, back, and chest. Use the truck as your prop to attach the bands.

(See figures.)

You can also go on YouTube to get other ideas for exercise that can be done in and around your truck.

Abdominal exercises are vital to your overall health, especially when you drive for so long. While driving, you can squeeze your abdominals and hold it for two minutes or the length of a song. Do this frequently throughout the day, at least once an hour.

Once you're parked, before the start of the day, do at least thirty sit-ups and build up to a hundred. Planks are also great. Wherever there is room, start off the exercise by getting on your hands and knees. Then place your forearms and hands on the bed in your cab. Move your legs back so that you are placing your weight on your toes. Try to make your body a straight line and hold for thirty to sixty seconds. (See pic.)

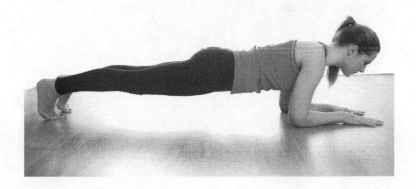

There is another great option for any of us, but especially truck drivers. It's called a Power Plate.

Power Plate is a vibration plate that vibrates twenty-five to fifty times per second, resulting in your muscles working much harder while exercising. This causes your muscles to contract much more than they would while doing regular exercise. Just standing on the plate with your knees slightly bent will increase muscle tone and strength. Different exercises can be done for the legs, arms, and abdomen.

The Power Plate also increases circulation and reduces edema or fluid buildup. It is low impact so that no matter what kind of shape you're in, you can do this. Bad knees? No problem. Back hurts? This will help. A cardio workout can be done with repetitions of lunges, press-ups, and sit-ups.

The vibration plate helps with muscle tone, strength, balance, and bone density; reduces visceral fat and cellulite; and increases metabolism on days of use. The plate also promotes healing of tendons and muscles.

The best vibration plate is the one called Power Plate at PowerPlate. com. (See pic.)

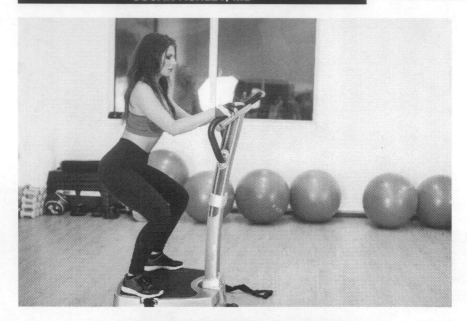

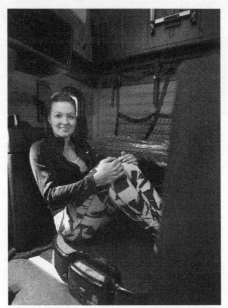

It is the only brand with the patented Tri-Planar vibration technology. It vibrates up and down, side to side, and front to back. Others typically only teeter-totter up and down and do not achieve the frequency and amplitude of the Power Plate. With Power Plate, wherever you make contact, all aspects of the vibration will be the same. Other products do not have the same quality and life span. The portable Power Plate is small, weighs about forty pounds, and can fit under the bed of your truck. It does need to be plugged in, which is not a problem for modern trucks. I recommend this brand without question. Go to PowerPlate.com.

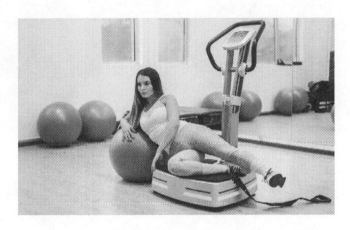

Section Six

Success

Chapter 31

Success

The key to success is to focus our conscious mind on things we desire and not things we fear.

—Brian Tracy.

What is the secret of success?

What would you do if you could do anything? If you could have any job, what would it be? If you could make any amount of money and be completely get out of debt? If you could have optimal physical health? If you could have a loving, fulfilling marriage and family? Impossible?

Absolutely not!

Realize that you have the spiritual DNA of God within you, and you have unlimited power. Most of us don't think of ourselves in this way. Instead, our thoughts are mostly negative, and this negativity is like bags of sand that weigh us down. The thoughts we think of ourselves are much more powerful than the thoughts that others think of us.

Every one of us is the sum total of our thoughts. You are where you are and doing what you're doing because that's exactly where you want to be, whether you admit it or not. What you think today and tomorrow will mold your life and determine your future. Every thought has a frequency that actually changes our brain waves and sends out a signal to the universe to attract these things. See yourself living in abundance, and you will attract abundance. See yourself living in poverty, paycheck to paycheck, and you will always live in poverty. You are affirming your debt and struggle.

This is called the law of attraction, and it is going on twenty-four hours a day.

Life is an adventure and should be lived at the fullest. You should want to get out of bed in the morning and be happy for the day that awaits you. The life you live is a reflection of the person you are and the thoughts that you dwell on. If you don't like this picture of your life, the first thing that must be done is to change your thoughts!

Grove Patterson, an editor for a major newspaper, once said, "People are basically good. We came from someplace, and we're going someplace, so we should make our time here an exciting adventure. The architect of the universe didn't build a stairway leading nowhere."

To become successful in this life, we must learn and believe that we literally become what we think about. We must control our thoughts if we are to control our lives. Any limits you think you have are limitations you put on yourself.

Most of us have heard the following Chinese proverb:

Watch your thoughts, they become words;
watch your words, they become actions;
watch your actions, they become habits;
watch your habits, they become character;
watch your character, for it becomes your destiny.

It all starts with our thoughts. You will become what you think about, and you attract to yourself what you dwell on. Look at the beauty and riches of the world and the abundance that is there. There is no reason why you can't have a part of it. It is not there only for someone else; it's there for you just as much as it is for them.

What I want you to do tonight, once you're done working for the day and are relaxing before bed, is to write down the things you would like in your life. And be specific. Don't just say "I want to be rich." Say exactly how much money you want in your bank account and by what time. Don't say "I want to be healthy." Say exactly how many pounds you are going to lose by a specific time. For thirty days, you will read your goals both during morning and night, and you will dwell on these goals. See yourself succeeding, and do not allow this picture to fade.

You must visualize the things you want, and see yourself already having them. Look at your life as if you've already achieved your dreams. By doing this daily, you'll notice things happening in your life that are bringing you closer to your goals.

I like to use a visualization board. Put pictures of the things you want on your board, and have this in your truck. Look at it in the morning and in the evening. Use this as a graphic illustration of what you want in life.

You are driving for hours a day, and you have a great opportunity to fill your mind with positive books and messages. Immerse yourself in audio books from the great authors in this area, authors such as

1. Norman Vincent Peale,
2. Napoleon Hill,
3. Zig Ziglar,
4. Joe Vitale,
5. Earl Nightingale,

6. Dale Carnegie,
7. Deepak Chopra,
8. Darrin Donnelly,
9. Bob Knight,
10. Denis Waitley,
11. Bob Proctor, and
12. Joel Osteen.

As you do this, you will find that you are changing. Your thoughts are changing, your habits are changing, your inspiration is changing, and your life is changing.

And don't worry! Worry is negative thinking that can be crippling, and when we worry about negative situations, we bring into our life the very things we don't want. We've been trained throughout life to doubt ourselves and to worry about things that never come to pass.

"You create your own universe" was said by Winston Churchill years ago, and it's as true then as it is now.

Fill your mind with positive affirmations, and repeat them throughout the day. Think thoughts such as the following:

- I am completely out of debt.
- Money flows to me easily and effortlessly.
- I have so much energy and abundant joy.
- My marriage is becoming stronger, deeper, and more fulfilling each day.
- People look up to me and see my worth; my confidence is soaring.
- I am in charge of how I feel today, and I choose happiness.
- My income is constantly increasing.
- I am grateful for a healthy body.
- I choose to be hopeful and optimistic.
- I am one of a kind.

- Today will be a gorgeous day!
- I am a money magnet and attract wealth and prosperity.
- All my problems have a solution.
- I love and approve of myself.
- I am determined and disciplined.
- I seek out the bright side in every situation.
- I am beautiful and smart and charming, and I naturally attract others to me.
- Perfect health is my divine right, and I claim it now.
- I am a child of the most high God, and I have the spiritual DNA of God.

There are many positive affirmations. Come up with your own. But don't put anything negative in the statement. For example, let's say you have a chronic pain in your leg. Instead of saying "I don't have pain in my leg anymore," say "My leg is healthy and strong and very comfortable." Instead of saying "I am not fat. I am not ugly," say "I am healthy, and I am beautiful (or handsome)."

An affirmative thought is a hundred times more powerful than a negative thought!

When you get the opportunity, watch the movie *The Secret*. It's on Netflix. It's a good review of many of these concepts.

Remember, God has put you here for a purpose. He gave you unique talents, ones you will need to reach your eternal destiny. Tap into those talents, and don't deny them. Life can be absolutely phenomenal, and it should be and will be.

Your future will be bright and limitless, whether it continues as a much-needed truck driver or any other career you have your heart set on.

I am thankful for you, for all truckers everywhere, for without you, our society could not continue to operate. Your job is often thankless, but I am thankful for everything you do.

I'd like to close with a poem by Emily Matthews:

Believe in Yourself
Believe in yourself—
in the power you have
to control your own life, day by day,
Believe in the strength
that you have deep inside,
and your faith will help
show you the way.

I want to help you, the truck driver, receive your optimal physical and mental health, and it is my hope that the information in these chapters will help you to do so. For more assistance, go to my website, TruckersGuidetoHealth.com. As a member of this community, you will receive free question-and-answer submissions. It's a blog where you can post useful information to help others, purchase high-quality supplements, receive a 10% discount on all purchases, and get help with exercise and diet. I hope to meet many of you on my site soon, and I look forward to hearing from you. In the meantime, don't give up on your path to a healthy and happy future!

Susan Ashley, MD